Spiritual Fitness In Ten Minutes A Day

Spiritual Fitness In Ten Minutes A Day

A 'get fit' course, guide and logbook

to chart your progress

MARGARET FOURIE

AND

ARTHUR G CLARKE

Library of Congress Control Number:		2010911573
ISBN:	Hardcover	978-1-4535-0327-0
	Softcover	978-1-4535-0326-3
	Ebook	978-1-4535-0328-7

Scripture taken from the HOLY BIBLE, NEW INTERNATIONAL VERSION®. Copyright© 1973,1978,1984 by International Bible Society. Used by permission of Zondervan Publishing House. All rights reserved.

The "NIV" and "New International Version" trade marks are registered in the United States Patent and Trademark Office by International Bible Society. Use of either trademark requires the permission of International Bible Society.

This book was printed in the United States of America.

To order additional copies of this book, contact:
Xlibris Corporation
0-800-644-6988
www.xlibrispublishing.co.uk
orders@xlibrispublishing.co.uk
300248

Contents

Spiritual fitness in 10 minutes a day

Have nothing to do with godless myths and old wives' tales; rather train yourself to be godly. For physical training is of some value, but godliness has value for all things, holding promise for both the present life and the life to come. 1 Timothy 4:7-8

Isn't it strange? We spend hours getting our bodies in shape, but very little time getting our souls in shape. That's what this spiritual fitness programme aims to do.

By 'spiritual fitness', we mean (1) training ourselves to live a holy life in a manner pleasing to God; and (2) becoming more alive to the wonder of our already existing union with God.

Surely, you will say, it takes more than 10 minutes a day to get spiritually fit! You're right. Growing spiritually fit is a full-time job. These 10 minutes—1% of your day—are dedicated recollection time when you give thanks for growth and reflect upon how you conducted your life that day.

You'll quickly discover your strengths and weaknesses and what you need to focus on.

The spiritual life should be a wondrous adventure, a great voyage of discovery. No particular talent or skill is needed to get started. All you need is a willing heart, some self-discipline, and the desire to love. Of course, in the end, it is God's grace working through you that will bring about the desired changes. By ourselves we can do nothing.

A STRUCTURED PROGRAMME

St Paul talks about the need for the spiritual person to 'train like an athlete' in order to be fit for God. Many runners keep logbooks. This is your spiritual logbook.

It will:

- measure your progress
- evaluate your relationship to God in six areas
- evaluate your relationship to your neighbour in three fields
- provide a daily meditation
- act as a journal and motivator to do better.

The goal is self-perfection—an impossible quest! But we can all make remarkable progress by becoming increasingly aware of God's presence in our lives night and day, by being good and doing good, by noticing how we think and act, and by reaching out to others.

We need to do everything for the glory of God.

We also need to avoid sin and selfishness—the major barriers to spiritual growth:

- the world (the inordinate love of material pleasures),
- the flesh (wrongful desires which harm us and lead us away from God),
- the devil (who lures and tempts us to rebel against God by committing acts that are unloving and unacceptable in His sight).

People are inclined to slip into bad habits and thought patterns. A ball dropped from a height bounces back again. A ball that gradually rolls down a slope stays at the bottom. By daily reviewing your situation, you are less likely to slide down that slippery slope.

The need for measurement

In all the important aspects of life, measurement takes place. But how does one measure spiritual fitness?

Within the realm of physical fitness, it's easy. Exercises are graded so that they become harder to do, increasing gradually in both difficulty and duration.

Within the realm of the spiritual life, a somewhat different technique is needed. We measure progress by the *effort expended* with the grace of God's help, rather than the *results achieved*.

How the programme works

Every evening, Monday to Saturday (Sunday is a day of rest) you will be asked to rate yourself that day on two questions. And then write down *in pencil*—a few words (not more than 11)—your answer to the meditation question that has been set for the day.

Scoring

You give yourself a score in two areas: (1) Your relationship with God; (2) Your relationship with your neighbour.

You score as follows:
8-10 (max): Excellent (did my best)
6-7: Good
5: Average
3-4: Fair
1-2: Poor (missed the mark hopelessly)

Your evaluations are subjective. The precise scores themselves are not the main thing. What matters is *the pattern of the scores*. Over time, you should find yourself scoring higher and higher marks. That's encouraging. God wants us to feel 'abundant joy' and we will feel this joy when we serve Him as we should.

The format is the same each week (although the questions change each day). Take a look at a typical week's training programme and then read the notes below.

In the example below, the symbol Ψ represents your relationship with God, the symbol ☺ represents your relationship with your neighbour. [M] is the symbol for Meditation.

WEEK 1 (& 14)

Did I . . .		Ψ	☺	TOTAL
Mon Date: Month:	001. Ψ . . . praise God for himself alone, and not only for his gifts? 002.☺ . . . do good? Encourage? Reduce stress? Bring out the best in others? [M] How can I make a better contribution? *Join a charity organization*	Prayer and Praise 7	Right action 4	11
Tues Date: Month:	003. Ψ . . . look for ways to love God and love my neighbour? 004.☺ . . . counter pessimistic views? Remain a centre of serenity? [M] What are my unused talents? *Good at listening sympathetically to others*	Faith and Friendship 6	Right attitude 7	13
Wed Date: Month:	005. Ψ . . . uphold God's ethical standards in my dealings? 006.☺ . . . avoid detraction, unseemly language? Refuse to bear a grudge? [M] When do I feel good about myself? *When I have really done my best—and praised!*	Discipline and discipleship 4	Right avoidance 3	7
Thur Date: Month:	007. Ψ . . . repent any unconfessed sins? Repent specific sins? 008.☺ . . . treat those who work for me as I would like to be treated? [M] Where do I find the greatest happiness? *Not sure—when completely involved with a project*	Repentance and renewal 4	Right action 8	12
Fri Date: Month:	009. Ψ . . . hear a word that seemed 'God inspired'? 010. ☺ . . . uplift the spirit? Consider others' unspoken needs? [M] Why do I want to grow in the spiritual life? *I want a deeper relationship with Jesus*	Learning and listening 3	Right attitude 6	9
Sat Date: Month:	011. Ψ . . . thank God for His constant love, care and friendship? 012.☺ . . . avoid pettiness, evil intents, thinking ill of others? [M] Who is able to help me grow spiritually? *Perhaps join a prayer group. Follow Joe's example*	Thanks and Trust 8	Right avoidance 8	16
	TOTAL WEEKLY SCORE	32	36	68

Sunday weekly journal:

_____

_____

_____

_____

More details about the daily programme

Each day you are asked three questions:

(1) Relationship with God [Ψ]

This is always the first question for the day and will draw your attention to one of the six categories shown below. Your score goes in the first column.

- **(a) Prayer and Praise**
  Praising and worshipping God.
- **(b) Faith and friendship**
  Deepening your relationship with our loving God.
- **(c) Discipline and discipleship**
  Doing those things that are pleasing to God.
- **(d) Repentance and renewal**
  Apologizing for sins and committing yourself to do better.
- **(e) Learning and listening**
  Study of the Bible or other religious books; hearing God's word in a number of ways.
- **(f) Thanks and trust**
  Thanking God and trusting in Him.

(2) Relationship with neighbour [☺]

This is always the second question for the day and will focus your attention on one of three categories. (Each of these three category questions appears twice a week.) Your score goes in the second column.

- **(a) Right action**
  What you have said or done to help, encourage and uplift others.
- **(b) Right attitude**
  What you have thought—your approach to others.
- **(c) Right avoidance**
  Negative or hurtful actions to be avoided.

Most evenings, on reflecting back, you should be able to find some actual experience during the day that relates to the daily questions asked. Occasionally, this may not be so. In this case, give yourself the score you think you would have got if the situation or circumstances depicted in the question had arisen.

Add your two scores together to get your total for the day.

(3) The meditation

This is always the third question for the day. Space has been provided for you to summarize your key thoughts in not more than a few words. All the questions start with the words: *who, what, when, where, why,* or *how.* As you progress spiritually, it will be useful to glance back at your meditations. (Should you finish your meditation early, there are supplementary meditation 'points to ponder' at the back of the book for each week.). Or meditate on one section of the Franciscan principles.

Sunday weekly journal

Sunday is a 'non-score' day of rest—a day for reflection, prayer and meditation. Space has been provided for you to jot down how you fared during the week. You may care to review your spiritual life over the last week as in the example below:

> *Main problem of week*: Shouting at spouse.
> *What was the occasion?* Accused of laziness.
> *What was the cause?* Conflict between watching sport on TV and doing the
>   shopping.
> *What do I resolve?* To listen to the message behind the accusation and
>   consider whether it is justified before responding.

You will find this journal of your spiritual life illuminating as the months go by.

The calendar year

The year has been divided into four quarters of thirteen weeks each. Questions for weeks 1-13 are repeated in weeks 14-26 to give you a chance to compare your scores between quarters in the *score charts at the back of the book.* (Getting spiritually fit should be fun.) Weeks 27-39 and weeks 40-52 are treated in a like manner.

Evaluating your progress

Each day, you can score a maximum of 10 points when evaluating yourself in either of the two areas: (1) Relationship with God' [Ψ] and (2) Relationship with Neighbour [☺]. Your daily maximum total is 20 points. Your score is based on how well **you** feel you have done that day. Don't feel bad if you score 'average' scores at first—you don't become a champion athlete overnight, nor a 'spiritual' champion!

Theoretically, your **weekly** maximum total score is:

6 days x 20 points = 120 points. (Sunday is a day of rest.)

For the sake of convenience, the **weekly** maximum scoring total in each of the *charts at the back of this book* has been limited to 100 points (or 100%). To achieve this weekly maximum score means you need to score just over 8.25 points on every single item for the entire week. If you manage to do this, you are either a saint—throw away this book!—or you over-evaluate your own contribution! The **total weekly score** represents your general success level that week. For some people this may be the only score they will want to keep, others will want to go further.

Using the charts

Three score charts have been provided for you at the back of this book:

(1) **Total weekly score:** A general review of your progress. Are you improving?
(2) **Comparative scores:** Which area are you doing best in?
(3) **Perseverance rating percentage.** How regularly are you doing your review sessions?

Here is an example of one of the score charts:

SPIRITUAL FITNESS SCORECARD
Table 1
WEEK'S TOTAL SCORE

Add together each week's totals under **God** and **Neighbour.** Note your weekly score with a dot and join with a line. Try to do better each quarter.

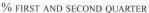

% FIRST AND SECOND QUARTER

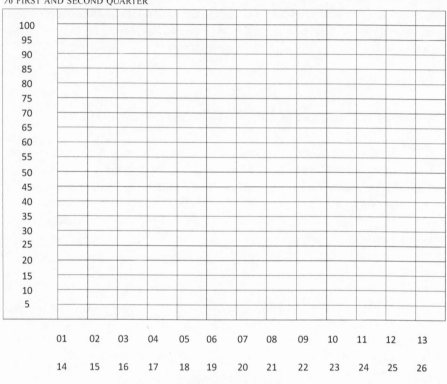

WEEKS

Using this book

- Do the exercises each day, and fill in your score.
- **A biblical quotation has been included for each question**, which may assist you. Refer to Biblical helps on page 122. They are numbered for your convenience. Tick off the ones that have been most helpful to you, and memorize them.
- Refer to page 165 to review your progress.
- Each Sunday review your week.

- Read through the 'training tips' and spiritual notes that accompany the weekly exercises.
- You will find a 'thanks' list and 'pray for' list at the back of this book.

Notes on the spiritual life

Many of us do not know too much about the spiritual life. We have provided a topic for you to think about each week that we hope you will find helpful. You can read these straight through. Or dip in here and there. Particularly you should read through these notes when God appears distant or absent, when your spiritual life is filled with aridity, or when your prayer life seems so much white noise bouncing off into space!

> . . . and let us run with perseverance the race marked out for us. Let us fix
> our eyes on Jesus, the author and perfecter of our faith . . . Hebrew 12.1-2

IMPORTANT!

While it is possible to score yourself and answer the questions set within a minute or two, don't do this! Give a full ten minutes to God each day. Ponder the biblical quotations provided. Really think carefully over your day, hour by hour, noting what you did well, and where you could have improved. Your time spent in careful and prayerful reflection and contemplation will put you on the right track in helping you to make rapid progress in the spiritual life. If you find yourself completing your review before the ten minutes is up, you can ponder on the 'attributes to cultivate' or 'sins to avoid' which have been set for that week, which you will find at the back of the book. Or simply remain silent before God.

Enjoy! God bless you.

A NOTE FOR CHURCH GROUP LEADERS AND PASTORS

This book has been designed primarily for use by individuals in the privacy of their own homes. Nevertheless, we believe it could prove a useful tool for members of weekly church 'cell groups'.

The questions have been designed to get people to look deeply into the way they put Christianity into practice in their lives. Many questions are sure to arise.

A cautionary note we think should be made. Unless the cell group members know each other extremely well and are prepared to share confidences at a deep level, we believe it is inadvisable to ask people what their precise scores were for the week. There is a great danger of spiritual pride and competitiveness creeping in which is most undesirable.

The aim should be to help people on their spiritual journey. The types of question the cell group leader can ask members of the group are:

- In which area did you score highest and lowest?
- Which did you find the most difficult question for you to answer?
- Which of the Biblical helps were most helpful?
- Did you learn something new about God this week?

Cell groups will probably easily be able to proceed from these starting points, with the cell group leader getting people to share their frustrations and difficulties, their learnings and insights.

Romans 8.6: It is death to limit oneself to what is unspiritual; life and peace can only come with concern for the spiritual. (Jerusalem Bible)

God never ceases to speak to us, but the noise of the world without and the tumult of our passions within bewilder us and prevent us from listening to him.

—F. Fénelon

Do all the good you can
By all the means you can
In all the ways you can
In all the places you can
To all the people you can
As long as ever you can.
—John Wesley

WEEK 1 (& 14)

Did I . . .		Ψ	☺	TOTAL
Mon Date: Month:	001. Ψ . . . praise God for himself alone, and not only for his gifts? 002.☺ . . . do good? Encourage? Reduce stress? Bring out the best in others? [M] How can I make a better contribution?	Prayer and Praise	Right action	
Tues — Date: Month:	003. Ψ . . . look for ways to love God and love my neighbor? 004.☺ . . . counter pessimistic views? Remain a centre of serenity? [M] What are my unused talents?	Faith and Friendship	Right attitude	
Wed Date: Month:	005. Ψ . . . uphold God's ethical standards in my dealings? 006.☺ . . . avoid detraction, unseemly language? Refuse to bear a grudge? [M] When do I feel good about myself?	Discipline and discipleship	Right avoidance	
Thur Date: Month:	007. Ψ . . . repent any unconfessed sins? Repent specific sins? 008.☺ . . . treat those who work for me as I would like to be treated? [M] Where do I find the greatest happiness?	Repentance and renewal	Right action	
Fri Date: Month:	009. Ψ . . . hear a word that seemed 'God inspired'? 010. ☺ . . . uplift the spirit? Consider others' unspoken needs? [M] Why do I want to grow in the spiritual life?	Learning and listening	Right attitude	
Sat Date: Month:	011. Ψ . . . thank God for His constant love, care and friendship? 012.☺ . . . avoid pettiness, evil intents, thinking ill of others? [M] Who is able to help me grow spiritually?	Thanks and Trust	Right avoidance	
	TOTAL WEEKLY SCORE			

Sunday weekly journal:

_____

_____

_____

_____

Spiritual Training programme
Week 1

Training tip

Your first task is to persevere in doing the exercises. No athlete gets fit by training only one day a week. It is the same with the spiritual life. Strive to do these exercises daily. Enjoy getting spiritually fit.

Words of encouragement
... Surely you will reward each person according to what he has done. Psalm 62:12

Perseverance points. Tick one block every day you do the exercises

1-10%	2-20%	3-40%	4-60%	5-80%	6-100%

WHY DO WE WANT TO BE HOLY?

The whole idea of seeking holiness seems a bit bizarre nowadays, when the emphasis is on indulgence rather than discipline; where the concept of delayed gratification is paid lip-service to, but not taken seriously.

Popular catchphrases, or advertising tag lines like 'Just do it!' 'I want it and I want it now!' 'If it feels good, do it' all seem to suggest that anyone who doesn't act like this has a screw loose.

Why *on earth* would anyone in the twenty-first century want to buck the trend and seek holiness?

Let's start by looking at what is meant by being holy. In the Old Testament the distinguishing feature is the concept of separation—in other words, not like the rest. This introduces a whole universe of thought. What is wrong with the rest? Why do we want to be different? Does this mean being isolated from the rest, lonely, or rejected? The short answer to that is 'No'—just the opposite in fact!

You have probably noticed how much corruption, greed, dishonesty, double standards, and violence there is in our society and our world today. We are also confronted with broken promises, broken marriage vows, broken lives. The very fabric of our society is tearing apart. Who should we trust?

So perhaps it is not such a bad idea to be different after all! Wanting to be holy involves being different from all this evil, as well as becoming a whole person—becoming truly human, made in the image of God himself. Is this what you want?

Thought for the week
If you love the sacred and despise the ordinary, you are still bobbing in the ocean of delusion. Lin-Chi

The whole essence of the spiritual life consists in recognizing the designs of God for us at the present moment. Jean-Pierre de Caussade

WEEK 2 (& 15)

Did I . . .		Ψ	☺	TOTAL
Mon Date: Month:	013. Ψ . . . live out my faith today? Build faith in others? 014. ☺ . . . make allowances for people acting under stress or ill health? [M] When do I feel most separated from God?	Faith and Friendship	Right attitude	
Tues Date: Month:	015. Ψ . . . maintain a right relationship with God? 016. ☺ . . . help someone? Pray for them? Act as a peacemaker? Thank? [M] What is my purpose in life?	Repentance and renewal	Right action	
Wed Date: Month:	017. Ψ . . . serve God by serving others? Support the church? 018. ☺ . . . avoid impatience, condescension, and hurting others? [M] Where do I most need to improve?	Discipline and discipleship	Right avoidance	
Thur Date: Month:	019. Ψ . . . pray with real belief that God hears and answers prayer? 020. ☺ . . . give pride of place to others? Give of myself? [M] Why do I believe in God?	Prayer and Praise	Right attitude	
Fri Date: Month:	021. Ψ . . . trust in God and accept his will for me without murmur? 022. ☺ . . . help my neighbour? Do something for my parents, family or children? [M] Who do I need to forgive?	Thanks and Trust	Right action	
Sat Date: Month:	023. Ψ . . . meditate on sacred scripture? 024. ☺ . . . avoid all aggression, gossip, and backbiting, blame? Bad-temper? [M] How do I become receptive to God's presence in my life?	Learning and listening	Right avoidance	
	TOTAL WEEKLY SCORE			

Sunday weekly journal:

_____

_____

_____

_____

Week 2

Training tip
Don't skimp on the 10 minutes you set aside each evening for your daily review session. Go through your day hour by hour. Athletes who focus on what they do make faster progress. So it is with spiritual athletes.

Words of encouragement
It is God's will that you should be sanctified. 1 Thessalonians 4:3

Perseverance points. Tick one block every day you do the exercises

1-10%	2-20%	3-40%	4-60%	5-80%	6-100%

DOING THINGS GOD'S WAY

Life is a gift. While we can do with it whatever we like, the question is: should we? Why bother to stick to the 'straight and narrow' if it means losing out? Why not watch pornographic movies—can there be any harm in that? Why give to the poor—they are not your problem, are they? Why be concerned about the other fellow? Is he or she concerned about you? Doesn't 'survival of the fittest' mean 'toughing it out' and getting what you want while you are young and fit enough to enjoy it?

What after all is the purpose of life?

For the Christian, the answer is quite clear: to glorify God. We are not our own. We belong to God. And God throughout the Bible and particularly through the example and words of his son Jesus has told us what he wants us to do and how we are to behave. We have been given commandments and counsels and some 40 parables, which show us how to act in certain situations. The Holy Spirit is ever present to help, guide and comfort us.

What then is our task? To be obedient to God and to do his will, following our Lord Jesus Christ who was obedient unto death. The task of obedience may be difficult at times—what worthwhile thing isn't?—but here's the strange part. You will find that the holiest people are not grim-faced, puritanical fanatics, but warm, happy, carefree, outgoing people who love life and others.

Thought for the week
Men are made for happiness, and anyone who is completely happy has a right to say to himself: "I am doing God's will on earth." Anton Chekhov

The spiritual is the parent of the practical. Carlisle

WEEK 3 (& 16)

Did I . . .		Ψ	☺	TOTAL
Mon Date: Month:	025. Ψ . . . offer my whole self to God holding nothing back? 026. ☺ . . . open someone's eyes to the beautiful, good, encouraging, amusing? [M] Where can I do most good?	Discipline and discipleship	Right action	
Tues Date: Month:	027. Ψ . . . give praise for His goodness, wisdom and infinite kindness? 028. ☺ . . . avoid all condescension, disparagement, undermining of another? [M] Why do I let other people upset me?	Prayer and Praise	Right avoidance	
Wed Date: Month:	029. Ψ . . . open myself to God's inspirations? 030. ☺ . . . ignore someone's failings and concentrate on their good? [M] When do I feel anxious or disquiet?	Learning and listening	Right attitude	
Thur Date: Month:	031. Ψ . . . give thanks to God for gifts given to others? 032. ☺ . . . avoid all deviousness, dogmatism, hypocrisy, unkindness, fault-finding? [M] Who do I pray for?	Thanks and Trust	Right avoidance	
Fri Date: Month:	033. Ψ . . . avoid self-delusion, covetousness, egotism, hypocrisy? 034. ☺ . . . show goodwill towards all? Forgiveness? Compassion? Follow our Lord's example? [M] How can I improve my prayer life?	Repentance and renewal	Right attitude	
Sat Date: Month:	035. Ψ . . . examine my motives for action before God, as my wise friend and counselor? 036. ☺ . . . befriend? lift other people's burdens? Go the extra mile? [M] What do I want out of life?	Faith and Friendship	Right action	
	TOTAL WEEKLY SCORE			

Sunday weekly journal:

_____

_____

_____

_____

Week 3

Training tip:
The big danger is quitting. In the scorecards you will find a section 'Perseverance rating and daily review.' Read the introductory pages again. Build your 'muscle memory' as to why you are doing the programme.

Words of encouragement

The LORD, the LORD, the compassionate and gracious God, slow to anger, abounding in love and faithfulness, maintaining love to thousands, and forgiving wickedness, rebellion and sin . . . Exodus 34:6,7

Perseverance points. Tick one block every day you do the exercises

1-10%	2-20%	3-40%	4-60%	5-80%	6-100%

THE JOY OF HOLINESS

Perhaps you are one of those people who say, 'Being holy? That's not me. I'm not that personality type. I can't be a priest or a monk or a nun. I'm not the introverted type who can lock myself away and spend hours and hours praying or fasting. I like the great outdoors, adventure, having fun!'

So do we!

The first thing to note is that God wants you to be uniquely you. We are not all the same, thank heavens. He wants you to enjoy life, to be filled with abundant joy. The truly holy person knows a joy that many other people don't. He or she becomes more receptive to others, to the grandeur and beauty of nature, to the miracles of life and death. Above all, the person who strives after holiness becomes more aware of God. God is not something 'out there'. God resides within, 'closer than the pulse of your neck'.

Sadly, the fact is that many of us don't notice him. He is not going to force himself down your throat. He invites you to him, to share with him all your frustrations and problems, to welcome you with loving arms, to offer you his transforming friendship, which will open your heart and mind to all the truly good things in life. And the truly good things in life are not money, fame and fortune, despite what some people say, but the love, joy and delight of knowing you are a child of God who loves you passionately.

Thought for the week

Sadness is a breath of hell; joy is the echo of God's life in us. Dom Marmion

Joy to the world! The Lord is come; let earth receive her King. Hymn

WEEK 4 (& 17)

Did I . . .		Ψ	☺	TOTAL
Mon Date: Month:	037. Ψ . . . confess my sins and failings without trying to hide anything? 038. ☺ . . . avoid complaining, indiscretions, or saying anything that dispirited? [M] What disturbs my equilibrium?	Repentance and renewal	Right avoidance	
Tues Date: Month:	039. Ψ . . . remain steadfast in the faith despite difficulties? 040. ☺ . . . approach others with consideration, care and compassion? [M] How has God helped me this day?	Faith and Friendship	Right attitude	
Wed Date: Month:	041. Ψ . . . thank God for opportunities to serve Him? 042. ☺ . . . reconcile differences? Cheerfully do a menial task? [M] Where do I lack self-control or self-understanding?	Thanks and Trust	Right action	
Thur Date: Month:	043. Ψ . . . look forward to my prayer times? 044. ☺ . . . help create a more stable situation? Fight injustice? Share a smile? [M] When should I pray?	Prayer and Praise	Right action	
Fri Date: Month:	045. Ψ . . . follow the precepts and counsels in Scripture? 046. ☺ . . . avoid moodiness, intrusion into others' privacy, attempts to dominate? Refrain from undermining authority? [M] Who else should I try to help?	Learning and listening	Right avoidance	
Sat Date: Month:	047. Ψ . . . put God first before everything else? 048. ☺ . . . set an example? Side with the weak and defenceless? [M] Why do I pray?	Discipline and discipleship	Right attitude	
	TOTAL WEEKLY SCORE			

Sunday weekly journal:

_____

_____

_____

_____

Week 4

Training tip
Always write a few words for your daily meditation. Thinking is tough! Get something down. Reminder: Each question has a number corresponding to a Biblical quotation starting on page 154.

Words of encouragement
Trust in the LORD with all your heart and lean not on your own understanding. Proverbs 3:5

Perseverance points. Tick one block every day you do the exercises

1-10%	2-20%	3-40%	4-60%	5-80%	6-100%

HOLINESS IS DOING GOD'S WILL

There is every reason to be holy. God is holy. Above all, he is love. To be holy is to be filled with God, which is to be filled with love. God's will for us is that we should love passionately and compassionately. It's as simple as that!

Jesus considered love so important that he summed up all religious teaching and the requirements of faith in two commands: love God with all your reason, all your emotions, all your actions and all your abilities; and love each other as much as you can love yourself. What a challenge! What an opportunity!

We all know that being in love and being loved in return is the best condition any human can be in. That is what God wills for us, not just for now but forever and ever. What heaven! Imagine the feeling you have when you love someone passionately and discover that they feel the same way about you—you feel beautiful, strong, wonderful, and above all, deliriously happy. Then imagine what it would be like to feel that for an eternity! Being with God, experiencing his love and being able to return it because he has made us holy, must be absolute heaven!

You cannot truly love what you do not know. That is why the person who strives after holiness spends so much time in study and prayer—building a relationship with God. Having God at the centre of your life, and willing what he wills, makes all the difference.

Thought for the week
If you lose the supernatural meaning of your life, your charity will be philanthropy; your purity, decency; your mortification, stupidity; your discipline, a lash; and all your works fruitless. Josemaria Escriva

WEEK 5 (& 18)

Did I . . .		Ψ	☺	TOTAL
Mon Date: Month:	049. Ψ . . . learn from the example/counsel of others? 050. ☺ . . . help others to find peace, perspective or overcome difficulties? [M] Why should I give my life to God?	Learning and listening	Right action	
Tues Date: Month:	051. Ψ . . . remain thankful and contented? 052. ☺ . . . avoid blaming, cold-shouldering, or slighting anyone? [M] How can I better cooperate with God?	Thanks and Trust	Right avoidance	
Wed Date: Month:	053. Ψ . . . pray for others with as much fervency as I pray for myself? 054. ☺ . . . cast aside remembered injuries? Take a firm stand when I saw injustice? [M] Who do I sometimes hurt, and how can I make amends?	Prayer and Praise	Right attitude	
Thur Date: Month:	055. Ψ . . . hold firmly to my faith? 056. ☺ . . . respond with love, really listening to the needs of others? [M] What virtues do I need to practice?	Faith and Friendship	Right attitude	
Fri Date: Month:	057. Ψ . . . wisely use my talents, treasure or time for His glory? 058. ☺ . . . avoid hassling, criticizing, embarrassing or interrupting others? [M] Where do I focus my attentions?	Discipline and discipleship	Right avoidance	
Sat Date: Month:	059. Ψ . . . run from temptation as from the face of a serpent? 060. ☺ . . . congratulate someone? Act with kindness? Alleviate someone's worries? [M] When am I resentful, self-serving or complacent?	Repentance and renewal	Right action	
	TOTAL WEEKLY SCORE			

Sunday weekly journal:

_____

_____

_____

_____

Week 5

Training tip

In any long-distance race you need the stamina that will keep you going until the very end. If we try to rely on our own strength we will always fail. Ask God to strengthen you.

Words of encouragement

When I called, you answered me; you made me bold and stouthearted. Psalm 138:3

Perseverance points. Tick one block every day you do the exercises

1-10%	2-20%	3-40%	4-60%	5-80%	6-100%

THE ROLE OF THE HOLY SPIRIT

All too often in our quest for 'spiritual perfection' we try to rely too much on ourselves. We are inclined to become full of ourselves and our own prowess, whereas we should be emptying ourselves and allowing God to work in us and through us.

The fact has to be faced that we cannot do it by ourselves. We shouldn't even try to do it by ourselves. The Holy Spirit will work powerfully in us if we will let him. There is nothing in life that cannot be used by the Holy Spirit to further our growth in faith, our wisdom in understanding, our love in action, our hope in salvation.

The Holy Spirit acts in a multitude of ways. Here are some. The Spirit gives life (*John 7:38*); gives gifts (*1 Corinthians 12*); counsels (*John 14:26*); strengthens and encourages (*Acts 9:31*); intercedes on our behalf (*Romans 8:26*); empowers (*Acts 1:8*).

Do we know when the Holy Spirit is at work in us? Sometimes yes, and palpably so. At other times, perhaps only with hindsight. For example, if you (say) gave money to a beggar, *barely recognising that you had done a good deed and quickly forgetting what you had done,* this virtually certainly was the work of the Holy Spirit in you—even though you won't realise it!

As a measure of your growth in the spiritual life, you should find yourself bearing the fruits of the Spirit. These are: love, joy, peace, patience, kindness, goodness, faithfulness, gentleness, and self-control (Galatians 5:22)

The Holy Spirit gives life. Be grateful and give thanks.

Thought for the week

It is the Spirit of God that must teach us Who Christ is and form Christ in us and transform us into other Christs. Thomas Merton

The goal of the spiritual life is the union of the soul with God by incessant conformity to the divine will. St Francis de Sales

WEEK 6 (& 19)

Did I . . .		Ψ	☺	TOTAL
Mon Date: Month:	061. Ψ . . . trust that God knows what is best for me? 062. ☺ . . . avoid situations in which my emotions could go astray? Avoid flattery? [M] Who is crying out for special attention and support?	Thanks and Trust	Right avoidance	
Tues Date: Month:	063. Ψ . . . apply any word of God to my life? Delight to do God's will? 064. ☺ . . . avoid tarnishing someone's dignity by speaking ill of others? [M] Why do I believe the Gospel?	Learning and listening	Right avoidance	
Wed Date: Month:	065. Ψ . . . have faith that with God all things are possible? 066. ☺ . . . thank someone for his or her good example? Build harmonious relationships? Help others? [M] How can I best eradicate my major faults?	Faith and Friendship	Right action	
Thur Date: Month:	067. Ψ . . . act in ways worthy of my Christian calling? 068. ☺ . . . act with prudence, justice, fortitude and temperance? [M] Where am I going—and why?	Discipline and discipleship	Right attitude	
Fri Date: Month:	069. Ψ . . . feel real sorrow for my own sins or saying anything nasty about others? 070. ☺ . . . assist the weak, despondent, those who feel unloved? [M] When am I inclined to over-react?	Repentance and renewal	Right action	
Sat Date: Month:	071. Ψ . . . pray for my enemies or those who have wronged me? 072. ☺ . . . treat someone I don't like with warmth and consideration? [M] What do I look forward to each day?	Prayer and Praise	Right attitude	
	TOTAL WEEKLY SCORE			

Sunday weekly journal:

_____

_____

_____

_____

Week 6

Training tip
Be honest. If you've done your best, give yourself 10 marks. Don't let false modesty creep in. Be a praiseworthy character and a doer of good deeds. Other spiritual gifts will follow.

Words of encouragement
Whoever serves me must follow me; and where I am, my servant will also be. John 12:26

Perseverance points. Tick one block every day you do the exercises

1-10%	2-20%	3-40%	4-60%	5-80%	6-100%

LOVE AND BE LOVED
The first point to remember about love is that you have a choice. It is simply not true to say, "I can't love". It may be enormously difficult, it may take some time to reach the point of being able to love, and to let your love grow like the mustard seed. The second point to remember is that love is not necessarily a wild, heart-palpitating passionate feeling. Many a time it is an act of will.

A daughter once had her aged mother move in with her. It was not long before there was tension in the house and our friend found that she was having difficulty loving her mother at all. She tried everything she could think of, but the irritation got worse. Finally she said to God, "I can't manage to love Mom, but I am willing for you to use me to love her." God then loved her mother through her, and she was able to behave, and then feel, quite differently. God does in us what we cannot do for ourselves, if we make ourselves available to him and are prepared to give him the freedom to change us.

Becoming a loving person takes practice. The Bible has a lot to say about love. Read 1 Corinthians 13:4-8 for a start. Read the Parable of the Good Samaritan (Luke 10:25-37). Above all, see how Jesus loved. Follow him.

The more you love, the more lovable you are, and the more others, in turn, will love you.

Thought for the week
Do all the good you can, in all the ways you can, to all the souls you can, in every place you can, at all the times you can, with all the zeal you can, as long as you can. John Wesley

Don't let your hearts grow numb. Albert Schweitzer

WEEK 7 (& 20)

Did I . . .		Ψ	☺	TOTAL
Mon Date: Month:	073. Ψ . . . say my prayers without haste or impatience? 074. ☺ . . . avoid making mountains out of molehills? Causing dissension? [M] How can I improve my relationships with others?	Prayer and Praise	Right avoidance	
Tues Date: Month:	075. Ψ . . . truly strive to live this day in a way pleasing to the Lord? 076. ☺ . . . go the extra mile to help someone? [M] When do I need to guard my tongue?	Discipline and discipleship	Right action	
Wed Date: Month:	077. Ψ . . . mark, learn or inwardly digest any words of Holy Scripture? 078. ☺ . . . remain peaceful? Show appreciation? [M] Why do I sometimes feel anxiety?	Learning and listening	Right attitude	
Thur Date: Month:	079. Ψ . . . thank and praise God for the kindnesses and help that others gave me? 080. ☺ . . . avoid acting mischievously, boring anyone with my troubles, resentment and anger? [M] What charities should I support?	Thanks and Trust	Right avoidance	
Fri Date: Month:	081. Ψ . . . repent unworthy thoughts? Guard my tongue? 082. ☺ . . . empathize with others? Help someone to relax? [M] Who at work needs my friendship?	Repentance and renewal	Right attitude	
Sat Date: Month:	083. Ψ . . . act as a faithful servant of God, doing good to all? 084. ☺ . . . Help promptly all who asked? Cheer people up? Listen? [M] Where has my behaviour been unchristian?	Faith and Friendship	Right action	
	TOTAL WEEKLY SCORE			

Sunday weekly journal:

_____

_____

_____

_____

Week 7

Training tip
Enjoy the process. It's not an exam. You'll have good days and bad days, good weeks and bad weeks. Be content to make gradual progress. Devotion and dedication are what God wants.

Words of encouragement
Whoever obeys his command will come to no harm, and the wise heart will know the proper time and procedure. Ecclesiastes 8: 5

Perseverance points. Tick one block every day you do the exercises

1-10%	2-20%	3-40%	4-60%	5-80%	6-100%

THINGS THAT MAKE HOLINESS DIFFICULT

Unfortunately, many factors may hinder us from achieving this happy state of holiness. We live in a fallen world in which our values and priorities have somehow gone wrong. There is the constant pressure to 'keep up with the Jones' and conform to the world's standards. For some, their religious education has been faulty and they have a wrong notion of who God is—a stern and autocratic taskmaster! Others see how poorly Christians sometimes behave and (rightly) feel no desire to follow such examples.

We may need to heal the scars of wrong done to us, to be cleansed from guilt for the wrongs we have done, or to eradicate bitterness and fear in our lives—all these are the work of God's Holy Spirit, the Spirit of love.

Our role in this life is to work with God in absolute trust, to believe and accept that he loves us despite our failings, to rely on him completely. This takes faith, patience, and courage—particularly when the going gets tough. Our aim should be to open ourselves to God for him to do in us what we can't do for ourselves—to make us holy.

One good place to start is to become aware of what barriers prevent us from allowing God to work his miracles in us:

    a.   The wrongful things we have done or are still doing (sins),
    b.   The things that have been, or are still being, done to us (injuries & hurts), and
    c.   The kinks in our personalities that seem to fall into neither group.

Thought for the week
I long to accomplish a great and noble task, but it is my chief duty to accomplish small tasks as if they were great and noble. Helen Keller

The capacity to care is the thing which gives life its deepest meaning and significance. Pablo Casals

WEEK 8 (& 21)

Did I . . .		Ψ	☺	TOTAL
Mon Date: Month:	085. Ψ . . . trustingly place all my difficulties in God's hands? 086. ☺ . . . avoid jumping to conclusions, imposing on anyone, behaving hurtfully? [M] When am I at my happiest and most relaxed?	Thanks and Trust	Right avoidance	
Tues Date: Month:	087. Ψ . . . accept fully that God forgives? Strive to do better? 088. ☺ . . . help those in trouble, sorrow, need, sickness? Instill hope? [M] What would I like to change?	Repentance and renewal	Right action	
Wed Date: Month:	089. Ψ . . . avoid being double minded or lukewarm? 090. ☺ . . . put others' wishes before my own? Look for the good? [M] Who do I need to share my spiritual life with?	Faith and Friendship	Right attitude	
Thur Date: Month:	091. Ψ . . . strive to be holy and temperate in thought, word and deed? 092. ☺ . . . help someone enjoy the day more? Solve someone's difficulties? [M] Why do I sometimes show off, boast or try to dominate?	Discipline and discipleship	Right action	
Fri Date: Month:	093. Ψ . . . pray with love, reverence and concentration? 094. ☺ . . . turn the other cheek? Minimize difficulties? Show goodwill? [M] How often do I read the psalms?	Prayer and Praise	Right attitude	
Sat Date: Month:	095. Ψ . . . hear the word of God and keep it? 096. ☺ . . . avoid dishonesty even though I could get away with it? Blaming others? [M] Where do I need to work harder?	Learning and listening	Right avoidance	
	TOTAL WEEKLY SCORE			

Sunday weekly journal:

_____

_____

_____

_____

Week 8

Training tip
Your scorecard at the back of the book provides a way to measure your spiritual fitness and progress. Examine your score in Table 2. Discern strengths and developmental areas.

Words of encouragement
Cast your bread upon the waters, for after many days you will find it again. Ecclesiastes 11:1

Perseverance points. Tick one block every day you do the exercises

1-10%	2-20%	3-40%	4-60%	5-80%	6-100%

FACING THE FACT OF SIN

In the Bible we discover a lot about sin—all those things that are less than perfect. There are an awful lot. The nature of sin is that it always destroys. It destroys our souls. It destroys our relationships. It ruins our peace of mind and sense of self-worth. It hurts others and ourselves. We cannot get away from that truth. "The wages of sin is death," says Scripture. (Romans 6:23) Not because God will punish us so much as because that is its very nature.

Holiness is related to wholeness—being healed from sin and its consequences.

Scott Peck speaks of marching to a different drum. Jesus, in the Sermon on the Mount (Matthew 5 & 6) turns received wisdom on its head and recommends exactly the opposite of what seems to be the way to achieve, to live successfully. He tells us that when we seek God's kingdom and its justice first, we will be better off than we could have imagined, not only in a spiritual sense, but in every part of our lives, practically, emotionally and mentally.

Sin is a word that is very unfashionable at the moment, largely because of how it has been used in an accusing way in the past. Most people are quite rightly against focusing on the negative, the failures. Judgementalism, that mindset which blames and finds fault, is responsible for a great deal of marginalisation, hurt and damage in people's lives. But sin is still the word we need to use.

Thought for the week
The sheep was not lost because it got in the thicket but because it had been separated from the shepherd. Arthur L. Miller

No matter how far you have gone on the wrong road, turn back.

WEEK 9 (& 22)

Did I . . .		Ψ	☺	TOTAL
Mon Date: Month:	097. Ψ . . . think and act the way Jesus would like? 098. ☺ . . . help others feel liked, happier and more joyful? Do my duty? [M] What would God have me do that I am not doing?	Discipline and discipleship	Right action	
Tues Date: Month:	099. Ψ . . . avoid distractions in prayer, or give them to God? 100. ☺ . . . avoid clinging to old animosities? Misinforming or manipulating anyone? [M] Where can I be more loving?	Prayer and Praise	Right avoidance	
Wed Date: Month:	101. Ψ . . . make any thanksgiving sacrifice to God? 102. ☺ . . . remain loyal to others, courteous and respectful to all? [M] Why do I not have a radical change of lifestyle?	Thanks and Trust	Right attitude	
Thur Date: Month:	103. Ψ . . . wait patiently for guidance? Really desire what I prayed for? 104. ☺ . . . avoid malicious gossip, dampening enthusiasm, mockery—even in fun? [M] Who can ensure that I am going about things the right way?	Repentance and renewal	Right avoidance	
Fri Date: Month:	105. Ψ . . . study with a meek, humble and teachable mind? 106. ☺ . . . do what I ought to do? Strengthen others? [M] When do I feel disinclined to turn to God?	Learning and listening	Right action	
Sat Date: Month:	107. Ψ . . . listen to the voice of conscience? 108. ☺ . . . think more of others than myself? Want their happiness? [M] How will I know when I have improved?	Faith and Friendship	Right attitude	
	TOTAL WEEKLY SCORE			

Sunday weekly journal:

_____

_____

_____

_____

Week 9

Training tip

Training is specific. Build on strengths, eliminate weaknesses. Muscles grow flabby from disuse. This training programme only works if you do. Missed a few days? No sweat. Start again.

Words of encouragement

Do not be anxious about anything, but in everything, by prayer and petition, with thanksgiving, present your requests to God. Philippians 4:6

Perseverance points. Tick one block every day you do the exercises

1-10%	2-20%	3-40%	4-60%	5-80%	6-100%

WHAT CAN WE DO ABOUT SIN?

In the New Testament, the Greek word used for sin is *hamartia*, which is an archery term meaning "missing the bull's eye"! So anything less than perfection in our behaviour comes under the heading of sin.

Does that make you want to give up before you have even started? It shouldn't, because *ultimately the responsibility for keeping us from sin belongs to God, and for him it is entirely possible.* Even in us!

The *first action* we need to take is to ask for the Holy Spirit to make us more Christ-like, to guide and guard us in thought, word and deed. The *second action* we need to take is to find forgiveness for past sins, both for those things we did displeasing to God, as well as for the good things we failed to do when we had the opportunity to do them. Confession involves identifying, admitting and naming our sins before God, and being sorry about them. (See also Week 27). The *third action* we need to take is to strive mightily to avoid sin and the occasions for sin. Easier said than done. We all go astray. We all at times prefer our own self-will to God's will. Our sins break God's heart. Remembering this, we will be more likely to "Flee from sin as from the face of a serpent," as St Francis de Sales advised.

A good sign of increasing holiness is when you become more and more aware of how often you fall short of God's impeccable standards.

Thought for the week

Our scientific power has outrun our spiritual power. We have guided missiles and misguided men. Martin Luther King, Jr

Destroy the seed of evil or it will grow up to your ruin. Aesop

WEEK 10 (& 23)

Did I . . .		Ψ	☺	TOTAL
Mon Date: Month:	109. Ψ . . . concentrate on things which are pure, lovely, good, virtuous? 110. ☺ . . . anticipate what needed to be done—and do it? [M] Who do I need to restore friendship with?	Repentance and renewal	Right action	
Tues Date: Month:	111. Ψ . . . trust God to guide me when I ask for his help? 112.☺ . . . apologize for upsetting anyone or for sowing discord? [M] When am I at my best?	Thanks and Trust	Right attitude	
Wed Date: Month:	113. Ψ . . . increase my faith by uniting with others? 114. ☺ . . . avoid overcharging, taking offence, making someone beholden to me? [M] Why do I go to Church?	Faith and Friendship	Right avoidance	
Thur Date: Month:	115. Ψ . . . practise a prayerful, methodical way of reading the Bible? 116. ☺ . . . avoid taking the credit for some action undeservedly? Avoid acting meanly? [M] How do I guard against vanity, envy or lust?	Learning and listening	Right avoidance	
Fri Date: Month:	117. Ψ . . . endure hardships willingly for Christ's sake? 118. ☺ . . . lead by example? Keep my promises? Act as a peacemaker? [M] What makes all the difference?	Discipline and discipleship	Right action	
Sat Date: Month:	119. Ψ . . . pray with attention, devotion, and humility? 120. ☺ . . . remain loyal? Remain upright and honest in all dealings? Help the oppressed? [M] Where is God trying to lead me?	Prayer and Praise	Right attitude	
	TOTAL WEEKLY SCORE			

Sunday weekly journal:

_____

_____

_____

_____

Week 10

Training tip
Some people may want to use the space for each Sunday to record prayer requests. They then tick off all requests that are fulfilled. Notice how God is working in and through you.

Words of encouragement
You may ask me for anything in my name [Jesus], and I will do it. John 14:14

Perseverance points. Tick one block every day you do the exercises

1-10%	2-20%	3-40%	4-60%	5-80%	6-100%

SIN AND GUILT

No one likes to feel guilty. Of course, if we keep our standards low enough, there is no problem whatever!

Yet some of us are all too conscious of one or more big, bad sins, and this tortures us with guilt. It is urgent that that sin be dealt with permanently immediately, that you receive full forgiveness for it so that it is no longer a huge mark on your conscience. It may be holding your attention off some other, deeper sins!

At home I have a pale cream-coloured carpet. Every so often I can no longer put up with the horrible marks on it and I get out the carpet stain-remover and set to work on the three or four big black marks. I work hard until they are gone. Then, as I sit back in triumph and admire my clean carpet, I notice eight or nine smaller black marks. I remove those. Once more I start to admire the carpet, only to become aware of dozens of blemishes. The first ones were so bad that I didn't notice the others. Each time I cleaned some, my standards for a clean carpet rose. So it is with the sin in our lives.

Guilt and shame, which accompany our wrong actions, are known to be very destructive and even express themselves in mental, physical and spiritual disease. The only function they have is to warn us that what we are doing is wrong. Once God has forgiven you, accept that forgiveness and *let go of the guilt forever.*

Thought for the week
No man chooses evil because it is evil; they only mistake it for happiness. Mary Wollstonecraft

In nature, nothing is perfect and everything is perfect. Trees can be contorted, bent in weird ways, and they're still beautiful. Alice Walker

WEEK 11 (& 24)

Did I . . .		Ψ	☺	TOTAL
Mon Date: Month:	121. Ψ . . . discover God through music, nature, art? 122. ☺ . . . sanctify all my actions? Search for the good in others? [M] Why should I do good if I would not be found out if I did wrong?	Learning and listening	Right attitude	
Tues Date: Month:	123. Ψ . . . lift up my soul in praise, thanks, and adoration? 124. ☺ . . . help the poor, the hungry, the lost, the lonely? [M] How do I cope with other people's difficulties?	Prayer and Praise	Right action	
Wed Date: Month:	125. Ψ . . . try to find an appropriate opportunity to 'preach the Gospel'? 126. ☺ . . . look upon others' faults with tolerance? Act with patience? [M] Who is lonely, troubled or longing for help?	Discipline and discipleship	Right attitude	
Thur Date: Month:	127. Ψ . . . realise what a deep and intimate relationship God wants with me? 128. ☺ . . . help around the home? Make everyone in my family feel loved? [M] What is God's greatest gift to me?	Faith and Friendship	Right action	
Fri Date: Month:	129. Ψ . . . thank God for his goodness? 130. ☺ . . . avoid dwelling on the faults of others, indifference, coldness, retaliation? [M] When do I become enthusiastic/?	Thanks and Trust	Right avoidance	
Sat Date: Month:	131. Ψ . . . resist evil? Keep all the Commandments? 132. ☺ . . . avoid someone's needs because I was too busy, tired, uncaring? [M] Where do I find strength in times of difficulty?	Repentance and renewal	Right avoidance	
	TOTAL WEEKLY SCORE			

Sunday weekly journal:

_____

_____

_____

_____

Week 11

Training tip
Remember that you are measuring the effort you put in. Sometimes our best actions do not bear fruit immediately. Relax! The best athletes have a relaxed style. God works with our sincere desire to please him.

Words of encouragement
Go, eat your food with gladness, and drink your wine with a joyful heart. Ecclesiastes 9:7

Perseverance points. Tick one block every day you do the exercises

1-10%	2-20%	3-40%	4-60%	5-80%	6-100%

THE MIRACLE OF FORGIVENESS

The good news is that God does not want us to carry a load of guilt, even if it is our own fault. He has gone to immense lengths to make it possible for us to be guilt-free, unashamed and happy. He is even more ready to forgive us than we are to ask!

After all, it is God who is at work in us, making us holy, and he above all others, understands us! The miraculous truth is that, once we have received forgiveness from God, it is as if what we had done had never happened (As far as the East is from the West, so far has he removed our transgressions from us—Psalm 103:12). Not only has he removed all the stain of sin, but we are also made completely innocent once more. (Though your sins are as scarlet, they shall be white a snow (Isaiah 1:18). If anyone is in Christ, they are a new creation (2 Corinthians 5:17)—i.e. innocent as the day you were born).

Does this mean that there are no consequences to sin? Suppose you were an alcoholic. Through God's grace once you realized the sinful way you were abusing your body, you prayed for forgiveness and reformed your way of life. Although the sin is forgiven, the damage to your body may have already been done. Sin has consequences.

Some of the exercises in this book may help you identify your sins and make it possible to bring them to God and receive his forgiveness.

Thought for the week
If you love, forgive, if you don't love, forget.

To err is human, to forgive, divine. Pope

WEEK 12 (& 25)

Did I . . .		Ψ	☺	TOTAL
Mon Date: Month:	133. Ψ . . . ask God to open my ears and my mind? 134. ☺ . . . encourage others by behaving cheerfully, calmly, bravely? [M] When do I prefer to give rather than receive?	Learning and listening	Right attitude	
Tue Date: Month:	135. Ψ . . . strive against blowing hot and cold, wavering or indecision? 136. ☺ . . . avoid disparaging someone because of his or her weight, dress, mannerisms? Avoid grumbling? [M] How do I retain a healthy lifestyle?	Faith and Friendship	Right avoidance	
Wed Date: Month:	137. Ψ . . . live blamelessly in the sight of God this day? 138. ☺ . . . help others not to act in a disruptive way? Calm troubled spirits? Promote peace and tranquillity? (M) Where do I lack self-discipline?	Repentance and renewal	Right action	
Thur Date: Month:	139. Ψ . . . trust God completely? 140. ☺ . . . act benevolently towards all? Forgive others? [M] What toxic thoughts do I hold?	Thanks and Trust	Right attitude	
Fri Date: Month:	141. Ψ . . . pray for the needs of communities and the world? 142. ☺ . . . avoid flirting, showing off, causing stress, meddling in others' affairs? [M] Why worry?	Prayer and Praise	Right avoidance	
Sat Date: Month:	143. Ψ . . . seek first the kingdom of God and his righteousness? 144. ☺ . . . give a smile to others? Do a charitable act? Listen? Cheer people up? [M] Who wants me to listen to them?	Discipline and discipleship	Right action	
	TOTAL WEEKLY SCORE			

Sunday weekly journal:

_____

_____

_____

_____

Week 12

Training tip
To strengthen our spiritual muscles we must constantly use them. Be careful not to grow introverted, watching yourself under the spotlight all the time. Let God do the work. Go with the flow.

Words of encouragement
I have swept away your offences like a cloud, your sins like a mist. Isaiah 44:22

Perseverance points. Tick one block every day you do the exercises

1-10%	2-20%	3-40%	4-60%	5-80%	6-100%

SIN AND RESTITUTION

Sometimes there are things you need to put right before you are able to receive God's forgiveness. We call 'putting matters right' acts of restitution. It may be to return what you have taken or to apologise for hurting someone. In a word, to make amends.

But take care. If, for instance, you have been unfaithful to your partner and he or she doesn't don't know about it, it may be immensely unkind to tell him or her in order to ease your own guilty conscience.

In a case like this, always check with your spiritual adviser before confessing to the person you have wronged—sometimes the sudden awareness of how they have been lied to or cheated may cause them immense pain. When someone else is involved, you certainly may not implicate that person without his or her consent. They will have to come to the point of penitence themselves. All you can do is confess your part of it, accepting responsibility for your own actions.

When you try to right wrongs, don't expect others to regard your actions as heroic! They may question the genuineness of your sorrow, or your sincerity or suspect you of an ulterior motive. Or make snide remarks behind your back that you are 'suffering from a guilty conscience'. Do not expect gratitude—people who have been wronged are often angry. Your sole reason in 'righting wrongs' should be because you know deeply in your heart, that this is what God wants you to do. Let love rule your life. Let your motives be pure.

Thought for the week
Always be a little kinder than necessary. James M. Barrie

If you want to meet a good person, do good things.

WEEK 13 (& 26)

Did I . . .		Ψ	☺	TOTAL
Mon Date: Month:	145. Ψ . . . pray even when I didn't feel like doing so? 146. ☺ . . . anticipate others' needs? Make someone feel valued? [M] Who really understands me?	Prayer and Praise	Right attitude	
Tues Date: Month:	147. Ψ . . . confess my sins and determine to amend with God's help? 148. ☺ . . . avoid worrying other people with my problems? Acting hurtfully? [M] What is my greatest fear?	Repentance and renewal	Right avoidance	
Wed Date: Month:	149. Ψ . . . apply any specific precepts to my life?? 150.☺ . . . do my duty? Return good for evil? [M] How have I grown as a Christian?	Learning and listening	Right action	
Thur Date: Month:	151. Ψ . . . truly believe that God is my loving Father? 152.☺ . . . act from pure motives or intentions? [M] Why do I not feel as happy or as peaceful as I would like?	Faith and Friendship	Right attitude	
Fri Date: Month:	153. Ψ . . . follow in the footsteps of Jesus in thought, word and deed? 154. ☺ . . . avoid arguing, being judgmental, snubbing others, nagging? [M] When am I likely to be impatient or lose my temper?	Discipline and discipleship	Right avoidance	
Sat Date: Month:	155. Ψ . . . thank God and remain cheerful? 156. ☺ . . . show gratitude? Patiently assist difficult people? [M] Where am I most selfish?	Thanks and Trust	Right action	
	TOTAL WEEKLY SCORE			

Sunday weekly journal:

_____

_____

_____

_____

Week 13

Training tip
You are now going to repeat the exercises you did in the first quarter. Your meditation answers may now be different. Time to start comparing scores. Make it your goal to beat your previous score.

Words of encouragement
Let us not become weary in doing good, for at the proper time we will reap a harvest if we do not give up. Galatians 6:9

Perseverance points. Tick one block every day you do the exercises

1-10%	2-20%	3-40%	4-60%	5-80%	6-100%

REPEATED SIN
What about when you confess your sin, are forgiven it, then go out and fall into it again?

Confess it again. Strive to do better. Sometimes it is difficult to get to the root cause of why we act as we do. A helpful approach here is not to concentrate on oneself and one's own sins, but on God, on his love and kindness, on his longing for you to constantly turn to him, on the deep relationship he wants with you.

People who are addicted (alcohol, cigarettes and drugs) battle terribly with the problem of 'repeated sins'. Yet how many of us waste our God-given lives addicted to computer games, watching sport, or the Internet. Other 'addictions' are more psychological such as the need for continual sexual gratification.

To deal with an addiction, you will need the help of someone else. You may find it in Alcoholics Anonymous, or Narcotics Anonymous or one of the other agencies of change. For other addictions, you will need to find a spiritual adviser or prayer partner to whom you will be accountable, and who will pray for you right throughout your period of recovery. Contact your priest or pastor, or your bible study leader, or one of the religious houses (convents, monasteries).

The good news is that, when you have been forgiven, that record of sin is expunged from your life, so that the next time, it is once again the *first time* you are doing it. Bring it to God and ask for forgiveness and strength once more.

Thought for the week
When with yourself watch your thoughts. When with others watch your speech.
Tibetan proverb

For anything worth having one must pay the price and the price is always work, patience, love, self-sacrifice. John Burroughs

WEEK 14 (& 1)

Did I . . .		Ψ	☺	TOTAL
Mon Date: Month:	001. Ψ . . . praise God for himself alone, and not only for his gifts? 002.☺ . . . do good? Encourage? Reduce stress? Bring out the best in others? [M] How can I make a better contribution?	Prayer and Praise	Right action	
Tues Date: Month:	003. Ψ . . . look for ways to love God and love my neighbor? 004.☺ . . . counter pessimistic views? Remain a centre of serenity? [M] What are my unused talents?	Faith and Friendship	Right attitude	
Wed Date: Month:	005. Ψ . . . uphold God's ethical standards in my dealings? 006.☺ . . . avoid detraction, unseemly language? Refuse to bear a grudge? [M] When do I feel good about myself?	Discipline and discipleship	Right avoidance	
Thur Date: Month:	007. Ψ . . . repent any unconfessed sins? Repent specific sins? 008.☺ . . . treat those who work for me as I would like to be treated? [M] Where do I find the greatest happiness?	Repentance and renewal	Right action	
Fri Date: Month:	009. Ψ . . . hear a word that seemed 'God inspired'? 010. ☺ . . . uplift the spirit? Consider others' unspoken needs? [M] Why do I want to grow in the spiritual life?	Learning and listening	Right attitude	
Sat Date: Month:	011. Ψ . . . thank God for His constant love, care and friendship? 012.☺ . . . avoid pettiness, evil intents, thinking ill of others? [M] Who is able to help me grow spiritually?	Thanks and Trust	Right avoidance	
	TOTAL WEEKLY SCORE			

Sunday weekly journal:

_____

_____

_____

_____

Week 14

Training tip
Every athlete suffers from aches and pains from time to time. It's part of the process. If you feel spiritually discomforted, be of good cheer. God loves you. Count your blessings.

Words of encouragement
Seek me and live. Amos 5:4

Perseverance points. Tick one block every day you do the exercises

1-10%	2-20%	3-40%	4-60%	5-80%	6-100%

THE IMPORTANCE OF FORGIVING OTHERS

To *receive forgiveness* for your sins, you also need *to forgive* others. Not forgiving others is one of the main obstacles to receiving forgiveness. Jesus says, "Forgive us our sins as we forgive those who sin against us." This doesn't mean that we have to forgive others in order to make God want to forgive us, like a prize for good behaviour—his forgiveness is free because Jesus has already paid the price. It is already there, waiting for us to ask for it and there is no qualification for it. The difficulty lies in whether or not we are able *to accept this forgiveness and forgive ourselves.* Learning to forgive others affects our own ability to receive forgiveness, just as learning to love helps us to be loved.

Caroline Myss once said that seeking revenge is like drinking poison and hoping that it kills the other person. If we withhold forgiveness because the other person "doesn't deserve it", we are acting very stupidly. We know that bitterness and resentment destroys human beings, so when we hold on to them, we see to it that the other person hurts us twice over, the second time by invitation!

Let go of anger and hurt and allow God to start the healing process. Hold on to Joel 2:25—read it now!—not only will he change your life, God's promises are greater: he will recompense you for all you lost because of what happened to you.

Thought for the week
I have found the paradox that if I love until it hurts, then there is no hurt, but only more love. Mother Theresa

If you hate a person, you hate something in him that is a part of yourself. What isn't part of ourselves doesn't disturb us. Herman Hesse

WEEK 15 (& 2)

Did I . . .		Ψ	☺	TOTAL
Mon Date: Month:	013. Ψ . . . live out my faith today? Build faith in others? 014. ☺ . . . make allowances for people acting under stress or ill health? [M] When do I feel most separated from God?	Faith and Friendship	Right attitude	
Tues Date: Month:	015. Ψ . . . maintain a right relationship with God? 016. ☺ . . . help someone? Pray for them? Act as a peacemaker? Thank? [M] What is my purpose in life?	Repentance and renewal	Right action	
Wed Date: Month:	017. Ψ . . . serve God by serving others? Support the church? 018. ☺ . . . avoid impatience, condescension, and hurting others? [M] Where do I most need to improve?	Discipline and discipleship	Right avoidance	
Thur Date: Month:	019. Ψ . . . pray with real belief that God hears and answers prayer? 020. ☺ . . . give pride of place to others? Give of myself? [M] Why do I want to be holy?	Prayer and Praise	Right attitude	
Fri Date: Month:	021. Ψ . . . trust in God and accept his will for me without murmur? 022. ☺ . . . help my neighbour? Do something for my parents, family or children? [M] Who do I need to forgive?	Thanks and Trust	Right action	
Sat Date: Month:	023. Ψ . . . meditate on sacred scripture? 024. ☺ . . . avoid all aggression, gossip, and backbiting, blame? Bad-temper? [M] How do I become receptive to God's presence in my life?	Learning and listening	Right avoidance	
	TOTAL WEEKLY SCORE			

Sunday weekly journal:

_____

_____

_____

_____

Week 15

Training tip
At the end of this week you will have completed the first quarter. Now is the time to complete all the score charts at the back of this training log.

Words of encouragement
May our Lord Jesus Christ himself and God our Father, who loved us and by his grace gave us eternal encouragement and good hope, encourage your hearts and strengthen you in every good deed and word. 2 Thessalonians 2: 16-17

Perseverance points. Tick one block every day you do the exercises

1-10%	2-20%	3-40%	4-60%	5-80%	6-100%

BLAMING SELF
Sometimes we are confused into thinking that we are totally responsible for the bad things that happen to us. True, some of our suffering **is** the consequence of our own sinful behaviour. Yet many people blame themselves for the sin of others. That is exactly what abusers want you to do. It lets them off being guilty if they can convince you that it was all your fault.

When we start to get closer to God, Satan doubles his efforts to dislodge our peace. One way he does this is to make us waste our time, grief and emotional energy on feeling bad when we have no need to. Satan loves to make us victims and slaves of our own distorted perceptions.

The secret is to know when we have sinned and when not. That is why we ask the Holy Spirit to cast his light into our lives. We then take time to thank him for victories won, for temptations resisted, for the holiness that is growing in us.

Behaving as if we are miserable worms all the time denies the work of the Spirit. It prevents us from giving praise and thanks for what God has achieved in us. Don't fall for the temptation to beat yourself up for others' evil. Ask for healing for the hurt you have experienced, for strength to forgive the person who has hurt you, and then confidently nestle into the arms of God who loves you to bits.

Thought for the week
Enlightenment means taking full responsibility for your life. William Blake

To dispose a soul to action we must upset its equilibrium. Eric Hoffer

WEEK 16 (& 3)

Did I . . .		Ψ	☺	TOTAL
Mon Date: Month:	025. Ψ . . . offer my whole self to God holding nothing back? 026. ☺ . . . open someone's eyes to the beautiful, good, encouraging, amusing? [M] Where can I do most good?	Discipline and discipleship	Right action	
Tues Date: Month:	027. Ψ . . . give praise for His goodness, wisdom and infinite kindness? 028. ☺ . . . avoid all condescension, disparagement, undermining of another? [M] Why do I let other people upset me?	Prayer and Praise	Right avoidance	
Wed Date: Month:	029. Ψ . . . open myself to God's inspirations? 030. ☺ . . . ignore someone's failings and concentrate on their good? [M] When do I feel anxious or disquiet?	Learning and listening	Right attitude	
Thur Date: Month:	031. Ψ . . . give thanks to God for gifts given to others? 032. ☺ . . . avoid all deviousness, dogmatism, hypocrisy, unkindness, fault-finding? [M] Who do I pray for?	Thanks and Trust	Right avoidance	
Fri Date: Month:	033. Ψ . . . avoid self-delusion, covetousness, egotism, hypocrisy? 034. ☺ . . . show goodwill towards all? Forgiveness? Compassion? Follow our Lord's example? [M] How can I improve my prayer life?	Repentance and renewal	Right attitude	
Sat Date: Month:	035. Ψ . . . examine my motives for action before God, as my wise friend and counselor? 036. ☺ . . . befriend? lift other people's burdens? Go the extra mile? [M] What do I want out of life?	Faith and Friendship	Right action	
	TOTAL WEEKLY SCORE			

Sunday weekly journal:

_____

_____

_____

_____

Week 16

Training tip
Why not set yourself a target of the total number of points you will obtain this week before your week starts? Go for it!

Words of encouragement
He gives strength to the weary and increases the power of the weak. Isaiah 40:29

Perseverance points. Tick one block every day you do the exercises

1-10%	2-20%	3-40%	4-60%	5-80%	6-100%

DEEPLY HIDDEN BARRIERS TO LOVING

Sometimes we find ourselves experiencing difficulties in loving because of something that is deep in our personality or psyche. Many of us have experiences buried deeply out of reach of our conscious minds. This may be because they are too horrible to handle, and our minds protect us from them. They still have an effect on our lives, however, and you will need to find healing for them before you can be really free. This may call for an expert, and there is a lot to be said for going to therapy with a Christian therapist or counsellor who is properly qualified to help you.

Sometimes we may have a condition that makes our spiritual growth difficult,—you may be bipolar, or depressed, schizophrenic or something similar, which requires medication. Get it. God has provided the medical fraternity with tremendous insight and skill in the treatment of many conditions, just so that we can find help when we need it.

Don't beat yourself up when the going is hard. Allow God to use all he has prepared for your help. Rest in him. Remember what the Psalmist tells us in Psalm 103: " . . . for he knows how we are formed, he remembers that we are but dust." God understands our difficulties and he is able to bring us through them in one way or another. Trust him and allow him to do the work for you.

The real barrier is not to believe that God wants your happiness. Happiness comes when you love God above all else.

Thought for the week
Not everything that is faced can be changed, but nothing can be changed until it is faced. James Baldwin

Everyone should carefully observe which way his heart draws him, and then choose that way with all his strength. Hasidic saying

WEEK 17 (& 4)

Did I . . .		Ψ	☺	TOTAL
Mon Date: Month:	037. Ψ . . . confess my sins and failings without trying to hide anything? 038. ☺ . . . avoid complaining, indiscretions, or saying anything that dispirited? [M] What disturbs my equilibrium?	Repentance and renewal	Right avoidance	
Tues Date: Month:	039. Ψ . . . remain steadfast in the faith despite difficulties? 040. ☺ . . . approach others with consideration, care and compassion? [M] How has God helped me this day?	Faith and Friendship	Right attitude	
Wed Date: Month:	041. Ψ . . . thank God for opportunities to serve Him? 042. ☺ . . . reconcile differences? Cheerfully do a menial task? [M] Where do I lack self-control or self-understanding?	Thanks and Trust	Right action	
Thur Date: Month:	043. Ψ . . . look forward to my prayer times? 044. ☺ . . . help create a more stable situation? Fight injustice? Share a smile? [M] When should I pray?	Prayer and Praise	Right action	
Fri Date: Month:	045. Ψ . . . follow the precepts and counsels in Scripture? 046. ☺ . . . avoid moodiness, intrusion into others' privacy, attempts to dominate? Refrain from undermining authority? [M] Who else should I try to help?	Learning and listening	Right avoidance	
Sat Date: Month:	047. Ψ . . . put God first before everything else? 048. ☺ . . . set an example? Side with the weak and defenceless? [M] Why do I pray?	Discipline and discipleship	Right attitude	
	TOTAL WEEKLY SCORE			

Sunday weekly journal:

_____

_____

_____

_____

Week 17

Training tip
The four R's: Review what you did. Repent of your mistakes and learn from them. Remind yourself of what God wants. Replace bad actions or thoughts with good ones.

Words of encouragement
Fight the good fight of faith. Take hold of the eternal life to which you were called . . . 1 Timothy 6:12

Perseverance points. Tick one block every day you do the exercises

1-10%	2-20%	3-40%	4-60%	5-80%	6-100%

UNLEARNING THE BAD HABITS

All of us will have to unlearn the bad habits of selfishness and fearfulness that we have constructed over the years. There is absolutely no value in hanging on to them. The exercises in this book will help you to be more aware of the areas that need your prayerful attention. Daily, ask God's Holy Spirit to develop new 'holy' habits in you.

It is an old Native American belief that there are two hungry wolves within each of us—one angry and vicious, the other loving and kindly. They constantly fight each other for mastery over our life. Which one will win? Why, the one you feed! God's Holy Spirit is constantly at work in us. But if we allow Satan a foothold, the battle to win us over has begun. We will become like our master. Whether Satan or God will win is entirely in our hands, insofar as we can decide whether we want to feed the thoughts, memories and urges from the one or the other. Through Jesus Christ it has now become possible for us to choose to feed the presence of God within us so that holiness will grow and thrive in us.

To get fit, we need the discipline of sticking to our exercise program. Results will follow automatically. Similarly, for the work of the Holy Spirit within us to bear fruit, we should act on the right spiritual food, and persevere. Then we are working with God, no longer blocking the holiness that it is his good pleasure to give us.

Thought for the week
Such as are your habitual thoughts, such also will be the character of your mind; for the soul is dyed by the colour of its thoughts. Marcus Aurelius

Great works are performed not by strength but by perseverance. Samuel Johnson

WEEK 18 (& 5)

Did I . . .		Ψ	☺	TOTAL
Mon Date: Month:	049. Ψ . . . learn from the example/counsel of others? 050. ☺ . . . help others to find peace, perspective or overcome difficulties? [M] Why should I give my life to God?	Learning and listening	Right action	
Tues Date: Month:	051. Ψ . . . remain thankful and contented? 052. ☺ . . . avoid blaming, cold-shouldering, or slighting anyone? [M] How can I better cooperate with God?	Thanks and Trust	Right avoidance	
Wed Date: Month:	053. Ψ . . . pray for others with as much fervency as I pray for myself? 054. ☺ . . . cast aside remembered injuries? Take a firm stand when I saw injustice? [M] Who do I sometimes hurt, and how can I make amends?	Prayer and Praise	Right attitude	
Thur Date: Month:	055. Ψ . . . hold firmly to my faith? 056. ☺ . . . respond with love, really listening to the needs of others? [M] What virtues do I need to practice?	Faith and Friendship	Right attitude	
Fri Date: Month:	057. Ψ . . . wisely use my talents, treasure or time for His glory? 058. ☺ . . . avoid hassling, criticizing, embarrassing or interrupting others? [M] Where do I focus my attentions?	Discipline and discipleship	Right avoidance	
Sat Date: Month:	059. Ψ . . . run from temptation as from the face of a serpent? 060. ☺ . . . congratulate someone? Act with kindness? Alleviate someone's worries? [M] When am I resentful, self-serving or complacent?	Repentance and renewal	Right action	
	TOTAL WEEKLY SCORE			

Sunday weekly journal:

_____

_____

_____

_____

Week 18

Training tip
Beware of the outward show. God looks into the heart. These exercises are not meant to be another of life's burdens. Enjoy the challenge. Simply do your best.

Words of encouragement
The Lord your God is with you, he is mighty to save. He will take great delight in you, he will quiet you with his love, he will rejoice over you with singing. Zephaniah 3:17

Perseverance points. Tick one block every day you do the exercises

1-10%	2-20%	3-40%	4-60%	5-80%	6-100%

THE BEST SPIRITUAL FOOD
When a baby is born, it can only digest the simplest of food, and it is best if it is fed with its mother's milk. As it grows, so it is able to take in and digest more and more complex foods, until it is able to eat a fully varied and balanced diet

So it is with us in our spiritual lives. At first when we come to know the Lord and to have him take over the control of our lives, we need a very specialized diet of encouragement and training. We need to be in a group studying the bible so that we get to familiarize ourselves with Scripture, and to know where to find help and information. We need to be in a regular fellowship where we can learn to worship and to pray. We need to hear regular preaching so that we get to understand the breadth of our faith, and the enormity of God's love for us.

As time goes on, we will still need to have that same input, but we may well find that God gradually lessens his miraculous encouragement and helps us to stand in faith; he may withhold the sense of his presence so that we learn to trust him in faith; he will allow us to encounter situations that allow us to receive his good gifts of patience, forgiveness, faithfulness and all those others that can only develop in difficult times.

Always we will need the precious food of the Lord's Supper, a means of grace and empowering spiritual food.

Thought for the week
I am born self-centred. And this is original sin. Thomas Merton

The Body of Christ given for you . . .

WEEK 19 (& 6)

Did I . . .		Ψ	☺	TOTAL
Mon Date: Month:	061. Ψ . . . trust that God knows what is best for me? 062. ☺ . . . avoid situations in which my emotions could go astray? Avoid flattery? [M] Who is crying out for special attention and support?	Thanks and Trust	Right avoidance	
Tues Date: Month:	063. Ψ . . . apply any word of God to my life? Delight to do God's will? 064. ☺ . . . avoid tarnishing someone's dignity by speaking ill of others? [M] Why do I believe the Gospel?	Learning and listening	Right avoidance	
Wed Date: Month:	065. Ψ . . . have faith that with God all things are possible? 066. ☺ . . . thank someone for his or her good example? Build harmonious relationships? Help others? [M] How can I best eradicate my major faults?	Faith and Friendship	Right action	
Thur Date: Month:	067. Ψ . . . act in ways worthy of my Christian calling? 068. ☺ . . . act with prudence, justice, fortitude and temperance? [M] Where am I going—and why?	Discipline and discipleship	Right attitude	
Fri Date: Month:	069. Ψ . . . feel real sorrow for my own sins or saying anything nasty about others? 070. ☺ . . . assist the weak, despondent, those who feel unloved? [M] When am I inclined to over-react?	Repentance and renewal	Right action	
Sat Date: Month:	071. Ψ . . . pray for my enemies or those who have wronged me? 072. ☺ . . . treat someone I don't like with warmth and consideration? [M] What do I look forward to each day?	Prayer and Praise	Right attitude	
	TOTAL WEEKLY SCORE			

Sunday weekly journal:

_____

_____

_____

_____

Week 19

Training tip
Growing 'spiritually fit' is a lifetime challenge. Among your circle of friends and acquaintances, try to find someone on whom to model your behaviour. But be yourself.

Words of encouragement
Be still before the LORD and wait patiently for him; do not fret when men succeed in their ways, when they carry out their wicked schemes. Psalm 37:7

Perseverance points. Tick one block every day you do the exercises

1-10%	2-20%	3-40%	4-60%	5-80%	6-100%

LET GOD SET THE PRIORITIES IN YOUR LIFE
Becoming holy has many steps, and we are not the ones to decide the order in which these are to come. God has his own sweet way of dealing with us, even though what he is doing may not be obvious on the outside.

For many of my younger years I was quite a heavy smoker. This did not go well with being a Methodist preacher and I prayed to be delivered. I had to admit that I was addicted and needed the grace of God in a miracle to set me free! For several years I prayed and nothing happened. God did not deliver me. I was heavily criticized but quite helpless without God's help. I could not understand why this was—although I was very blessed in other ways. It was only after many years that I was delivered, and now, looking back I can see that God was working on other deeper and more dangerous things that were hidden, like spiritual pride. That would have sent me to hell long before smoking, which was a continual embarrassment In fact, having to constantly confront my own weakness and helplessness was a great help—I could never ever think of myself as better than anyone else, and everyone round me knew it!

So don't get discouraged. God ALWAYS answers your prayers. Jesus himself tells us in Luke 11:13 that God really loves to give us his Spirit to do in us what we cannot do for ourselves.

Thought for the week
You find yourself refreshed by the presence of cheerful people. Why not make earnest efforts to confer that pleasure on others? Half the battle is gained if you never allow yourself to say anything gloomy. L. M. Child

Love, and do what you will. St Augustine

WEEK 20 (& 7)

Did I . . .		Ψ	☺	TOTAL
Mon Date: Month:	073. Ψ . . . say my prayers without haste or impatience? 074. ☺ . . . avoid making mountains out of molehills? Causing dissension? [M] How can I improve my relationships with others?	Prayer and Praise	Right avoidance	
Tues Date: Month:	075. Ψ . . . truly strive to live this day in a way pleasing to the Lord? 076. ☺ . . . go the extra mile to help someone? [M] When do I need to guard my tongue?	Discipline and discipleship	Right action	
Wed Date: Month:	077. Ψ . . . mark, learn or inwardly digest any words of Holy Scripture? 078. ☺ . . . remain peaceful? Show appreciation? [M] Why do I sometimes feel anxiety?	Learning and listening	Right attitude	
Thur Date: Month:	079. Ψ . . . thank and praise God for the kindnesses and help that others gave me? 080. ☺ . . . avoid acting mischievously, boring anyone with my troubles, resentment and anger? [M] What charities should I support?	Thanks and Trust	Right avoidance	
Fri Date: Month:	081. Ψ . . . repent unworthy thoughts? Guard my tongue? 082. ☺ . . . empathize with others? Help someone to relax? [M] Who at work needs my friendship?	Repentance and renewal	Right attitude	
Sat Date: Month:	083. Ψ . . . act as a faithful servant of God, doing good to all? 084. ☺ . . . Help promptly all who asked? Cheer people up? Listen? [M] Where has my behaviour been unchristian?	Faith and Friendship	Right action	
	TOTAL WEEKLY SCORE			

Sunday weekly journal:

_____

_____

_____

_____

Week 20

Training tip
Athletes face headwinds, tough terrain, steep climbs, easy passages. It's the same with your spiritual life. Make all these up and downs an exciting challenge. Simply do your best each day.

Words of encouragement
The salvation of the righteous comes from the LORD; he is their stronghold in time of trouble. Psalm 37:39

Perseverance points. Tick one block every day you do the exercises

1-10%	2-20%	3-40%	4-60%	5-80%	6-100%

BELIEVE AND TRUST
We have to decide whether or not we really believe in God. I am sure that everyone reading this book would say, "Of course I believe in God!" but it may be salutary to remember that Satan himself also believes in God. The real question is: Do you believe and trust in God? We so often behave as if God were not real; as if God were not truly alive and involved in our world and in our lives.

How many times have you not been with Christian folk who are in a panic about something? How many times have you not found in yourself that you can't, for instance, live with uncertainty, because you "need to know so that I can plan"? The only reason you could have for needing so badly to know the future is so that you can try to prevent harm from coming, or try to provide for yourself or your loved-ones. Of course God has given us intelligence to foresee and forestall many difficulties and you should use these. But when the way is dark and uncertain there is no need to panic. Remember that you are not solely responsible for the well-being of your family. You have a partner in God!

None of us can *ultimately* control what happens to us in life. (We're only one heartbeat away from death!) Always remember that God is in charge. It is one of the great tests of our identity as Christians: trusting in God absolutely.

Thought for the week
A moment of choice is a moment of truth. Stephen R. Covey

It is not certain that everything is uncertain. Blaise Pascal

WEEK 21 (& 8)

Did I . . .		Ψ	☺	TOTAL
Mon Date: Month:	085. Ψ . . . trustingly place all my difficulties in God's hands? 086. ☺ . . . avoid jumping to conclusions, imposing on anyone, behaving hurtfully? [M] When am I at my happiest and most relaxed?	Thanks and Trust	Right avoidance	
Tues Date: Month:	087. Ψ . . . accept fully that God forgives? Strive to do better? 088. ☺ . . . help those in trouble, sorrow, need, sickness? Instill hope? [M] What faults do I need to eradicate?	Repentance and renewal	Right action	
Wed Date: Month:	089. Ψ . . . avoid being double minded or lukewarm? 090. ☺ . . . put others' wishes before my own? Look for the good? [M] Who do I need to share my spiritual life with?	Faith and Friendship	Right attitude	
Thur Date: Month:	091. Ψ . . . strive to be holy and temperate in thought, word and deed? 092. ☺ . . . help someone enjoy the day more? Solve someone's difficulties? [M] Why do I sometimes show off, boast or try to dominate?	Discipline and discipleship	Right action	
Fri Date: Month:	093. Ψ . . . pray with love, reverence and concentration? 094. ☺ . . . turn the other cheek? Minimize difficulties? Show goodwill? [M] How often do I read the psalms?	Prayer and Praise	Right attitude	
Sat Date: Month:	095. Ψ . . . hear the word of God and keep it? 096. ☺ . . . avoid dishonesty even though I could get away with it? Blaming others? [M] Where do I need to work harder?	Learning and listening	Right avoidance	
	TOTAL WEEKLY SCORE			

Sunday weekly journal:

_____

_____

_____

_____

Week 21

Training tip
At times, we all find it difficult to be of good cheer, or to praise God whole-heartedly or to love our neighbour. The desire to be our best self for God's glory is not without reward.

Words of encouragement
This is what the LORD says—your Redeemer, the Holy One of Israel: I am the LORD your God, who teaches you what is best for you, who directs you in the way you should go. Isaiah 48:17.

Perseverance points. Tick one block every day you do the exercises

1-10%	2-20%	3-40%	4-60%	5-80%	6-100%

THE PRACTICE OF FAITH MAKES PERFECT

As a priest, I have often heard people say, "If only I had your faith." Yes, faith is a gift from God. Let us give thanks for that. God gives each of us the degree of faith we need in this life to carry out his good purposes.

Part of the challenge of faith is to struggle through difficulties, to cling to biblical truths when our world seems to be collapsing around us, to carry on "carrying on". Faith is the acorn that grows into the mighty oak, if we will let it grow.

Some people may say, "I don't have enough faith to do this or that". The question is: Why not? Why do you have more faith in your doubts than faith in faith? Where has God ever let you down?

In the Lord's Prayer, you will have prayed time and again: "Thy will be done". The question is: do you mean this? Very often we only want God's will to be done if we can recognise it as one of our own identified range of options. Read Psalm 37 and take heart. Read 2 Chronicles 20—the battle is his and he will act!

It is the practice of our faith that increases it, in the same way that exercise increases muscle strength. Practising your faith means allowing God to lead you in situations where you cannot see the solution, and then resting in the love of God, waiting for him to act.

Pray for the faith to understand this.

Thought for the week
Faith is the bird that feels the light and sings when the dawn is still dark. Rabindranath Tagore

If we pray, we will believe; If we believe, we will love; If we love, we will serve. Mother Theresa

WEEK 22 (& 9)

Did I . . .		Ψ	☺	TOTAL
Mon Date: Month:	097. Ψ . . . think and act the way Jesus would like? 098. ☺ . . . help others feel liked, happier and more joyful? Do my duty? [M] What would God have me do that I am not doing?	Discipline and discipleship	Right action	
Tues Date: Month:	099. Ψ . . . avoid distractions in prayer, or give them to God? 100. ☺ . . . avoid clinging to old animosities? Misinforming or manipulating anyone? [M] Where can I be more loving?	Prayer and Praise	Right avoidance	
Wed Date: Month:	101. Ψ . . . make any thanksgiving sacrifice to God? 102. ☺ . . . remain loyal to others, courteous and respectful to all? [M] Why do I not have a radical change of lifestyle?	Thanks and Trust	Right attitude	
Thur Date: Month:	103. Ψ . . . wait patiently for guidance? Really desire what I prayed for? 104. ☺ . . . avoid malicious gossip, dampening enthusiasm, mockery—even in fun? [M] Who can ensure that I am going about things the right way?	Repentance and renewal	Right avoidance	
Fri Date: Month:	105. Ψ . . . study with a meek, humble and teachable mind? 106. ☺ . . . do what I ought to do? Strengthen others? [M] When do I feel disinclined to turn to God?	Learning and listening	Right action	
Sat Date: Month:	107. Ψ . . . listen to the voice of conscience? 108. ☺ . . . think more of others than myself? Want their happiness? [M] How will I know when I have improved?	Faith and Friendship	Right attitude	
	TOTAL WEEKLY SCORE			

Sunday weekly journal:

_____

_____

_____

_____

Week 22

Training tip
Turn constantly to God. Believe that he wants to help you. Notice those areas (Table 2) where you have scored the highest and lowest marks. Make gradual improvement your aim.

Words of encouragement
I will lead the blind by ways they have not known, along unfamiliar paths I will guide them; I will turn the darkness into light before them and make the rough places smooth. Isaiah 42:16

Perseverance points. Tick one block every day you do the exercises

1-10%	2-20%	3-40%	4-60%	5-80%	6-100%

THE EYES OF FAITH

When we speak about the "eyes of faith" we are talking about a way of living, an orientation, a way of viewing the world. People often speak about regarding a half-glass of water as either half full or half empty, the first being an optimistic, positive way of looking at things and the second a negative, pessimistic view.

In the same way, we can see things and thus experience our lives either through the eyes of the world, (cynical, suspicious and self-interested), or we can see things through the eyes of faith, which is an entirely different view.

Yes, there is pain and ugliness in the world. But also good things and beauty. The crucial question that each person must decide for himself or herself is this: is God in charge? The Christian, despite the difficulties and contradictory evidence that may surface, says, "Yes—I believe in God. I believe he is loving and good. I believe his infinite intelligence transcends my puny intellect and questionings."

Through the eyes of faith, we see the vast possibilities built into each situation—even painful disappointments, apparent disasters and tragedies, in God's hands, can be used as the raw materials for something worthwhile. When you have to endure pain, don't waste it. It is too costly for you to allow it to produce only negative results in you. Allow God to direct you through it and support you in it, and to create, gradually, something of beauty. Isaiah 61:3 reminds us of what God can do.

Thought for the week
Christ: the life of the soul.—Book title

Truly, spiritual obedience is to do through faith in the Son of God what you are ordered to do by God's command. Luther

WEEK 23 (& 10)

Did I . . .		Ψ	☺	TOTAL
Mon Date: Month:	109. Ψ . . . concentrate on things which are pure, lovely, good, virtuous? 110. ☺ . . . anticipate what needed to be done—and do it? [M] Who do I need to restore friendship with?	Repentance and renewal	Right action	
Tues Date: Month:	111. Ψ . . . trust God to guide me when I ask for his help? 112. ☺ . . . apologize for upsetting anyone or for sowing discord? [M] When am I at my best?	Thanks and Trust	Right attitude	
Wed Date: Month:	113. Ψ . . . increase my faith by uniting with others? 114. ☺ . . . avoid overcharging, taking offence, making someone beholden to me? [M] Why do I go to Church?	Faith and Friendship	Right avoidance	
Thur Date: Month:	115. Ψ . . . practise a prayerful, methodical way of reading the Bible? 116. ☺ . . . avoid taking the credit for some action undeservedly? Avoid acting meanly? [M] How do I guard against vanity, envy or lust?	Learning and listening	Right avoidance	
Fri Date: Month:	117. Ψ . . . endure hardships willingly for Christ's sake? 118. ☺ . . . lead by example? Keep my promises? Act as a peacemaker? [M] What makes all the difference?	Discipline and discipleship	Right action	
Sat Date: Month:	119. Ψ . . . pray with attention, devotion, and humility? 120. ☺ . . . remain loyal? Remain upright and honest in all dealings? Help the oppressed? [M] Where is God trying to lead me?	Prayer and Praise	Right attitude	
	TOTAL WEEKLY SCORE			

Sunday weekly journal:

_____

_____

_____

_____

Week 23

Training tip
To go deeper. You are encouraged to buy books that will show you the various pathways that the Christian saints have taken during their time here on earth.

Words of encouragement
For the LORD your God is the one who goes with you to fight for you against your enemies and to give you victory. Deuteronomy 20:4

Perseverance points. Tick one block every day you do the exercises

1-10%	2-20%	3-40%	4-60%	5-80%	6-100%

THE IMPORTANCE OF PRAYER

Since God knows our every thought and need, why does God ask us to pray constantly, and with faith? God knows and loves us, so why do we need to keep on telling him what we want him to do?

Of course we don't need to tell God what to do! But we do need to talk to him about our hopes and dreams, our fears for ourselves and others, and for many other reasons. We should feel free to talk to him about everything that is on our minds. The most important reason why we need to do this is to maintain contact . . . to embrace him.

Prayer is a conversation with God. And conversation is meant to go both ways. We talk to him and he listens to us. He talks to us and we listen to him. Unfortunately, most of us are not very good listeners, not so? How poor is that relationship if one person always only addresses the other with a list of 'I wants'. Building a relationship, with God or with anyone else, means lots of time spent together, lots of sharing thoughts and ideas, not merely speaking of wants and needs. God is our friend. If you, in your relationships with other people were continually to keep saying, "I want", that relationship wouldn't last very long, would it? You can see that there's something rather immature and selfish in acting this way.

Prayer is making yourself available to God, enjoying him, wanting to be with him.

Thought for the week
Our prayers are answered, not when we are given what we ask, but when we are challenged to become what we could be.

If you want to grow in the spirit of prayer, forget about "spiritual exercises" as things to be done. Think of them as personal tributes of love and loyalty . . . a seeking for a more intimate personal knowledge of Father, Son and Spirit. E.J Cuskelly

WEEK 24 (& 11)

Did I . . .		Ψ	☺	TOTAL
Mon Date: Month:	121. Ψ . . . discover God through music, nature, art? 122. ☺ . . . sanctify all my actions? Search for the good in others? [M] Why should I do good if I would not be found out if I did wrong?	Learning and listening	Right attitude	
Tues Date: Month:	123. Ψ . . . lift up my soul in praise, thanks, and adoration? 124. ☺ . . . help the poor, the hungry, the lost, the lonely? [M] How do I cope with other people's difficulties?	Prayer and Praise	Right action	
Wed Date: Month:	125. Ψ . . . try to find an appropriate opportunity to 'preach the Gospel'? 126. ☺ . . . look upon others' faults with tolerance? Act with patience? [M] Who is lonely, troubled or longing for help?	Discipline and discipleship	Right attitude	
Thur Date: Month:	127. Ψ . . . realise what a deep and intimate relationship God wants with me? 128. ☺ . . . help around the home? Make everyone in my family feel loved? [M] What is my best attribute I can use for God?	Faith and Friendship	Right action	
Fri Date: Month:	129. Ψ . . . thank God for his goodness? 130. ☺ . . . avoid dwelling on the faults of others, indifference, coldness, retaliation? [M] When do I become enthusiastic/?	Thanks and Trust	Right avoidance	
Sat Date: Month:	131. Ψ . . . resist evil? Keep all the Commandments? 132. ☺ . . . avoid someone's needs because I was too busy, tired, uncaring? [M] Where do I find strength in times of difficulty?	Repentance and renewal	Right avoidance	
	TOTAL WEEKLY SCORE			

Sunday weekly journal:

_____

_____

_____

_____

Week 24

Training tip
Are you scoring yourself too harshly? Too leniently? As we grow in perfection, we begin to see how far we fall short of real perfection. Be kind to yourself.

Words of encouragement
The LORD will keep you from all harm—he will watch over your life. Psalm 121:7

Perseverance points. Tick one block every day you do the exercises

1-10%	2-20%	3-40%	4-60%	5-80%	6-100%

WHY WE SHOULD PRAY
If we are to get to know God and to allow him into our hearts and to work deep within us, then we need to spend lots of time with him, sharing our thoughts and ideas, feelings and doubts, and sometimes, just being with Him, just as true lovers can sit in contented silence being with one another.

The main reason we have for praying is simply because God is. Our thoughts are drawn to him all through the day, in admiration and wonder. In addition to our more formal times of prayer, there is the constant conversation that takes place in the background of all the things that occupy us. We grow increasingly aware that in God we have a guiding presence, a loving friend, a comforter, and encourager.

In any prayerful life there is usually a great deal of praise. Whenever we get close to God, we find ourselves overcome with wonder, and the urge to praise him. Scripture tells us that God dwells in the praise of his people. Whenever you feel far away from God, praising him is one of the best ways to come close once more. One way of doing this is to think of different names for God (as many as you can)—Almighty, Creator, Father, All-knowing, Saviour, the Merciful and so on. Using your hymnal can also help with praising.

We need to pray so that we remain constantly aware of him and his presence in our lives. How else will we ever be able to recognize his voice?

Thought for the week
Prayer is not an old woman's idle amusement. Properly understood and applied, it is the most potent instrument of action. Gandhi

Don't ask for things to get better, ask that YOU get better. Jim Rohn

WEEK 25 (& 12)

Did I . . .		Ψ	☺	TOTAL
Mon Date: Month:	133. Ψ . . . ask God to open my ears and my mind? 134. ☺ . . . encourage others by behaving cheerfully, calmly, bravely? [M] When do I prefer to give rather than receive?	Learning and listening	Right attitude	
Tue Date: Month:	135. Ψ . . . strive against blowing hot and cold, wavering or indecision? 136. ☺ . . . avoid disparaging someone because of his or her weight, dress, mannerisms? Avoid grumbling? [M] How do I retain a healthy lifestyle?	Faith and Friendship	Right avoidance	
Wed Date: Month:	137. Ψ . . . live blamelessly in the sight of God this day? 138. ☺ . . . help others not to act in a disruptive way? Calm troubled spirits? Promote peace and tranquillity? (M) Where do I lack self-discipline?	Repentance and renewal	Right action	
Thur Date: Month:	139. Ψ . . . trust God completely? 140. ☺ . . . act benevolently towards all? Forgive others? [M] What toxic thoughts do I hold?	Thanks and Trust	Right attitude	
Fri Date: Month:	141. Ψ . . . pray for the needs of communities and the world? 142. ☺ . . . avoid flirting, showing off, causing stress, meddling in others' affairs? [M] Why worry?	Prayer and Praise	Right avoidance	
Sat Date: Month:	143. Ψ . . . seek first the kingdom of God and his righteousness? 144. ☺ . . . give a smile to others? Do a charitable act? Listen? Cheer people up? [M] Who wants me to listen to them?	Discipline and discipleship	Right action	
	TOTAL WEEKLY SCORE			

Sunday weekly journal:

_____

_____

_____

_____

Week 25

Training tip
Never give up. Have faith. Determine that you will improve. Now may be a good time to go over your answers to your meditation questions.

Words of encouragement
Delight yourself in the LORD and he shall give you the desires of your heart. Psalm 37:4

Perseverance points. Tick one block every day you do the exercises

1-10%	2-20%	3-40%	4-60%	5-80%	6-100%

PRAISE AND THANKSGIVING

Remember, when you are praising God that praise is not quite the same as thanksgiving, though they do support each other. Praise is really about enjoying God for who he is, and soaking in his splendour. What may surprise you is the degree to which your spirits lift when you start praising. Try praising for a couple of weeks and see for yourself. The order of Morning Prayer is almost all praise.

But there is more to prayer than just praising God. There is also thanksgiving. Merlyn Carrothers, in his books about praise, writes of the way we can express our trust in God by thanking him for things as they are, and not always asking him to change them. In fact, if we don't even have to decide what is good in the situation, but thank God for it as it is anyway, we have begun to trust him completely. Keep reminding yourself, "God knows about this!"

There is an old chorus that was popular in the last century:
> Count your blessings, name them one by one;
> Count your blessings, see what God has done:
> Count your blessings, name them one by one,
> And it will surprise you what the Lord has done.

It would be most wonderful if we could have that same attitude about all the things that happen to us—so often what looks like a disaster today turns out to be a blessing in disguise, when we look back after a while!

Thought for the week
It is a beauteous evening, calm and free,
The holy time is quiet as a Nun
Breathless with adoration . . . Wordsworth

No duty is more urgent than that of returning thanks. St. Ambrose

WEEK 26 (& 13)

Did I . . .		Ψ	☺	TOTAL
Mon Date: Month:	145. Ψ . . . pray even when I didn't feel like doing so? 146. ☺ . . . anticipate others' needs? Make someone feel valued? [M] Who really understands me?	Prayer and Praise	Right attitude	
Tues Date: Month:	147. Ψ . . . confess my sins and determine to amend with God's help? 148. ☺ . . . avoid worrying other people with my problems? Acting hurtfully? [M] What is my greatest fear?	Repentance and renewal	Right avoidance	
Wed Date: Month:	149. Ψ . . . apply any specific precepts to my life?? 150.☺ . . . do my duty? Return good for evil? [M] How have I grown as a Christian?	Learning and listening	Right action	
Thur Date: Month:	151. Ψ . . . truly believe that God is my loving Father? 152.☺ . . . act from pure motives or intentions? [M] Why do I not feel as happy or as peaceful as I would like?	Faith and Friendship	Right attitude	
Fri Date: Month:	153. Ψ . . . follow in the footsteps of Jesus in thought, word and deed? 154. ☺ . . . avoid arguing, being judgmental, snubbing others, nagging? [M] When am I likely to be impatient or lose my temper?	Discipline and discipleship	Right avoidance	
Sat Date: Month:	155. Ψ . . . thank God and remain cheerful? 156. ☺ . . . show gratitude? Patiently assist difficult people? [M] Where am I most selfish?	Thanks and Trust	Right action	
	TOTAL WEEKLY SCORE			

Sunday weekly journal:

_____

_____

_____

_____

Week 26

Training tip
Sometimes in any training programme there seem to be periods when we are not making progress. Simply persevere. Right effort always has its recompense in the long run.

Words of encouragement
Wait for the LORD; be strong and take heart and wait for the LORD. Psalm 27:14

Perseverance points. Tick one block every day you do the exercises

1-10%	2-20%	3-40%	4-60%	5-80%	6-100%

PRAYER AIDS

Many useful aids are available to help you. One is your prayer book. In most prayer books there is a wealth of wonderfully composed prayers that you can use. Even in denominations that do not have liturgical worship, there is usually some book of prayers for special occasions, and some liturgy for the Eucharist (Communion). Use this as a springboard for your own prayers. Look up the prayers written by others—they've had many of the same experiences as you and have been able to reflect on them. Try saying these prayers softly aloud—it really helps. Or sit down and compose the most beautifully crafted prayer you can which expresses your most genuine and deepest feelings.

Another useful aid is the hymn book, especially one of the new ones. There are a number of excellent hymns written from the depth of human experience, and these will enable you to praise and reflect on God in many different ways. This is not to ignore the great value of the older hymn books, in which we find great hymns that have stood the test of time, and deep theology and help for virtually any of life's situations. We often sing words without thinking about what we are saying. Reading hymns without the tune can open a treasure trove of devotional aids.

Then, of course, there are the Psalms: of praise, of longing and pain, of the whole human condition. Even the angry psalms remind us that we can be honest with God—he can cope with all our emotions!

Thought for the week
Children are God's apostles, day by day
Sent forth to preach love and hope, and peace. James Russell Lowell

Use what language you will, you can never say anything but what you are. Emerson

WEEK 27 (& 40)

Did I . . .		Ψ	☺	TOTAL
Mon Date: Month:	157. Ψ . . . behave in a way pleasing to him? Rely on God completely? 158. ☺ . . . create contentment rather than discontent? Share a smile? [M] When do I feel closest to God?	Repentance and renewal	Right attitude	
Tues Date: Month:	159. Ψ . . . praise God in all His majesty? 160 ☺ . . . give of my time, money, energy or talent to help others? [M] Why do I sometimes feel depressed? What should I do about it?	Prayer and Praise	Right action	
Wed Date: Month:	161. Ψ . . . do what Jesus would have me to do—despite difficulties? 162. ☺ . . . refrain from childishness, recklessness? Avoid prejudice? [M] How do I show I love God?	Discipline and discipleship	Right avoidance	
Thur Date: Month:	163. Ψ . . . have faith in God's holy laws? 164. ☺ . . . avoid becoming over-anxious? Avoid behaving rashly? [M] Where are opportunities for me to do good?	Faith and Friendship	Right avoidance	
Fri Date: Month:	165. Ψ . . . ask for divine inspiration before starting to study God's word? 166. ☺ . . . exercise compassion expecting nothing in return? [M] What energises me?	Learning and listening	Right attitude	
Sat Date: Month:	167. Ψ . . . act as a trusty steward in the position that God placed me? 168. ☺ . . . say something to make people feel that they mattered? Empathize? [M] Who is my neighbour?	Thanks and Trust	Right action	
	TOTAL WEEKLY SCORE			

Sunday weekly journal:

_____

_____

_____

_____

Week 27

Training tip
Congratulations. You have reached the halfway mark on your year's journey. Time to examine your scores over the last six months. Enjoy the challenge. As you start this second six months, make sure you know your strengths and weakness through analysis of your scores.

Words of encouragement
Blessed are all who fear the LORD, who walk in his ways. You will eat the fruit of your labor; blessings and prosperity will be yours. Psalm 128:1-2

Perseverance points. Tick one block every day you do the exercises

1-10%	2-20%	3-40%	4-60%	5-80%	6-100%

CONFESSION AND FORGIVENESS
Part of prayer often needs to be about confession and receiving God's forgiveness. What is important to know—really to know—is that God has already forgiven us for everything, that we can find complete freedom from guilt in a moment. The difficulty comes in being able to *receive* this forgiveness, and to forgive ourselves as well. Forgiveness from God does not come on its own. It is part of the relationship we can have with our Lord. Part of our interaction with God is that we become horribly aware of just how much of our lives is nasty, disappointing, shameful and grubby. Part of our interaction is also coming to understand how much God wants us to be free from the shame and guilt, and to perceive something of the sheer joy of being made whole.

We claim the forgiveness of God by being ruthlessly honest about ourselves, our motives and our lives, and by allowing God's Spirit to get to work in us, changing us. But just as it is hard to love others if you hate yourself, so it is impossible to receive forgiveness from God unless you learn to forgive others. Not forgiving others cuts you off from experiencing the wonder of God's transforming love.

This means not holding grudges, not keeping a record of someone else's faults, not needing to find out whose fault it is, who to blame. It means apologizing to others, being really sorry—sorry enough to accept the release and joy of being truly forgiven!

Thought for the week
As the circle of light grows, so does the circumference of darkness around it.
Albert Einstein

Confession is an act of self-accusation because it is the actual telling of what we have done wrong. It is not a simple admission of guilt nor a mere act of confidence in God's mercy. Catholic Catechism

WEEK 28 (& 41)

Did I . . .		Ψ	☺	TOTAL
Mon Date: Month:	169. Ψ . . . read the Bible or other religious texts prayerfully, carefully and remain open to the truth? 170. ☺ . . . avoid being self-righteous? Avoid being presumptuous and swollen-headed? [M] Where is God?	Learning and listening	Right Avoidance	
Tues Date: Month:	171. Ψ . . . strive for purity of heart? Avoid inordinate desires? 172. ☺ . . . give alms, a gift, or courage to others? Cheer anyone up? [M] When am I a good listener?	Repentance and renewal	Right action	
Wed Date: Month:	173. Ψ . . . examine the causes of, or reasons for, any doubts? 174. ☺ . . . try to understand others' needs, tastes, frustrations, hopes? Reach out? [M] Why do I not have a vision for my life? (if I don't)	Faith and Friendship	Right attitude	
Thur Date: Month:	175. Ψ . . . say 'flash prayers' during the day for others? 176. ☺ . . . behave with hospitality? Help the underprivileged? [M] How do I practice self-denial?	Prayer and Praise	Right action	
Fri Date: Month:	177. Ψ . . . do what God wanted, acting diligently at all times? 178. ☺ . . . give more than would be expected from common decency? [M] Who do I dislike most—and why?	Discipline and discipleship	Right attitude	
Sat Date: Month:	179. Ψ . . . conclude my prayers with thanks? 180. ☺ . . . avoid comparisons with another? Refrain from being petty? [M] What are my best and worst qualities?	Thanks and Trust	Right avoidance	
	TOTAL WEEKLY SCORE			

Sunday weekly journal:

_____

_____

_____

_____

Week 28

Training tip
You are now moving on to a completely different set of questions. What areas need special attention? Where do you find the greatest difficulty? What have you learned? Champion athletes think about what they are doing.

Words of encouragement
And all these blessings will come upon you and accompany you if you obey the LORD your God. Deuteronomy 28:2

Perseverance points. Tick one block every day you do the exercises

1-10%	2-20%	3-40%	4-60%	5-80%	6-100%

WORKING PROBLEMS THROUGH WITH GOD
Prayer gives us a chance to work through issues with God, and for him to help us into a different frame of mind. What we should be striving for is to put on the mind of God. Sometimes what we are asking for seems wonderful at the time, but might be a disaster later on.

Liesl was four when she prayed "Dear Lord Jesus, please will you make sweeties get bigger in my mouth when I suck them, instead of smaller." God did not grant her request!

Sometimes it is only after we have prayed for something for a long time that we begin to realize that we are praying for something that would not be helpful. This is particularly so when we pray for God to change someone else. When we pray, it is useful to spend some time in silence so that God can speak through our thoughts and direct our understanding.

Many of us may have tried asking that question "What would Jesus do?" (if he were in my shoes). That's often helpful. You might want to try also asking, "What wouldn't Jesus do?"

Sometimes it may be a good idea simply to say, "God—please help", and then wait. At other times it may be useful to sit down at your computer and have a long conversation with God in which you type out your question and write down what you imagine God would say in response. Often as you do this you will find that matters become much clearer.

And then, time and again, God uses others to help us. So don't be afraid to ask.

Thought for the week
Try to smile lovingly at every manifestation of God's will. Dom Marmion.

As it is with the earth so with the garden of our souls there is a winter that comes before the springtime. It is necessary. Dom Marmion

WEEK 29 (& 42)

Did I . . .		Ψ	☺	TOTAL
Mon Date: Month:	181. Ψ . . . pray meaningful and not empty words? 182. ☺ . . . behave sensitively? Make sure I did not cause offence? [M] How can I be of more service to others? ⬚	Prayer and Praise	Right attitude	
Tues Date: Month:	183. Ψ . . . meditate on God's precepts? 184. ☺ . . . renounce inordinate self-love? Renounce my own will? [M] Where do I do my best work? ⬚	Learning and listening	Right avoidance	
Wed Date: Month:	185. Ψ . . . trust God to answer my prayers? 186. ☺ . . . pay debts promptly? Thank? Treat others generously? [M] When am I most truly 'myself'? ⬚	Thanks and Trust	Right action	
Thur Date: Month:	187. Ψ . . . strive mightily to eradicate faults as well as ask for God's help? 188. ☺ . . . avoid letting others get me down through negative talk? [M] Who dislikes me—and why? ⬚	Repentance and renewal	Right avoidance	
Fri Date: Month:	189. Ψ . . . believe that God wants to be my friend? 190. ☺ . . . give, do or say something unexpectedly nice for someone? [M] What is it I really love and why? ⬚	Faith and Friendship	Right action	
Sat Date: Month:	191. Ψ . . . endure sufferings or difficulties with patience? 192. ☺ . . . strive to be a blessing to others? ? Listen with care rather than foster my own opinion on others? [M] Why am I doing these exercises? ⬚	Discipline and discipleship	Right attitude	
	TOTAL WEEKLY SCORE			

Sunday weekly journal:

_____

_____

_____

_____

Week 29

Training tip
We are commanded to love God, neighbour and self. The scores enable you to see how you put your love of God and your neighbour into practice. The daily meditation enables you to understand yourself better.

Words of encouragement
Have I not commanded you? Be strong and courageous. Do not be terrified; do not be discouraged, for the LORD your God will be with you wherever you go. Joshua 1:9

Perseverance points. Tick one block every day you do the exercises

1-10%	2-20%	3-40%	4-60%	5-80%	6-100%

ASKING
There are often times when we need help, or when there is something we dearly want. Jesus tells us to believe that we have what we pray for (Mark 11:24), so if we truly believe and trust in God, and that God wants us to have this good, we will pray with the visualization of the answer already in our mind's eye. All too often people pray for something and then with a lame sigh say "Thy will be done" which may be an indication that they don't really believe God would approve of what they ask for, or that God answers heartfelt prayer.

Sheila had a worn passage carpet and there was no prospect of finding the money in the budget to replace it. I suggested she ask God for one. She was shocked. "You can't ask God for a new passage carpet", she said. "Why not?" I asked. "Because God has much more important things to worry about."

The miracle is that God, while he does have the entire world in his hands, cares about Sheila's passage as well, and loves to give his darlings gifts. There is nothing you cannot ask God for. Of course, it is up to him whether or not he says yes, but you may certainly speak to him about whatever is on your mind.

Apart from material wants, ask for spiritual gifts too. Pray for more kindness, more patience, more love, and a deeper faith. Or pray that you may be used as the instrument for sharing God's goodness with others.

Thought for the week
"Who is there?" asks God. "It is I." "Go away," God says.
Later . . . "Who is there?" asks God. "It is thou." "Enter," replies God.

But all shall be well and all shall be well and all manner of thing shall be well. Julian of Norwich.

WEEK 30 (& 43)

Did I . . .		Ψ	☺	TOTAL
Mon Date: Month:	193. Ψ . . . have faith in God's goodness rather than material wealth? 194. ☺ . . . let my Christian conviction shine forth? Forgive and forget? [M] Where do I find peace?	Faith and Friendship	Right attitude	
Tues Date: Month:	195. Ψ . . . say grace before meals? Ask blessings for others? 196. ☺ . . . avoid self-indulgence? Gluttony? Wayward behaviour? [M] What Christian attributes do I lack?	Prayer and Praise	Right avoidance	
Wed Date: Month:	197. Ψ . . . practise detachment from things? 198. ☺ . . . refuse to cover up blind spots in my moral and spiritual life? [M] Who is a source of temptation for me?	Repentance and renewal	Right avoidance	
Thur Date: Month:	199. Ψ . . . stick to my Bible reading plan? 200. ☺ . . . say kindly words? Share a smile? Congratulate? Make amends? [M] When do I feel most compassionate?	Learning and listening	Right action	
Fri Date: Month:	201. Ψ . . . give thanks for all things? Rely on Him completely? 202. ☺ . . . listen with care? Speak truthfully? Refrain from anger or bearing grudges? [M] How do I prevent stress, negativity or despondency?	Thanks and Trust	Right attitude	
Sat Date: Month:	203. Ψ . . . purge bad dispositions? Act in the right way from the right motives? 204. ☺ . . . treat all with kindness? Stand up for the faith? Say a good word? [M] Why do I pray for peace when the world is continually at war?	Discipline and discipleship	Right action	
	TOTAL WEEKLY SCORE			

Sunday weekly journal:

_____

_____

_____

_____

Week 30

Training tip
Are you using the "prayer list" and "thanks" list on pages 142 and 144 to ensure that you regularly pray for a wide number of people and give thanks often?

Words of encouragement
Open wide your mouth and I will fill it. Psalm 81:10

Perseverance points. Tick one block every day you do the exercises

1-10%	2-20%	3-40%	4-60%	5-80%	6-100%

WHY KEEP ON AND ON ASKING?

Asking for something is called petition. It may be something for ourselves or for someone else. Yet if God knows all about us, why do we have to keep asking him?

One of God's special people in Cape Town, the late Ruth Cook, once asked God why she should go on and on praying for the same thing—it was rather like nagging and she felt it was rude. In response God gave her a vision of the situation she had been praying for, his grace and power shining like a beam of light towards it and a high brick wall in-between blocking the light. As she prayed, one brick loosened.

The simple answer is because that is what he wills for us to do. He encourages us time and time again to ask. It is not that God wants us to become totally subservient and dependent on him—we are anyway!—but He wants us to turn constantly to him because he is our very life. Persistence and perseverance in most things pay dividends, and help to establish 'holy habits'. It's the same with prayer.

Another reason is that sometimes it is only when we speak our minds that we obtain clarity as to what it is we exactly want.

Whether the situation is one within yourself, or something outside your life—even a national or international event—keep praying and allow God to use your faithful prayers to loosen the bricks of the dividing wall.

Thought for the week
Fear him, you saints, and you will then
Have nothing else to fear.
Make you his service your delight—
He'll make your wants his care
          -Nahum Tate & Nicholas Brady

WEEK 31 (& 44)

Did I . . .		Ψ	☺	TOTAL
Mon Date: Month:	205. Ψ . . . trust God sufficiently to avoid anxiety? 206. ☺ . . . listen patiently? Give my full attention to someone with a problem? [M] Why serve God if it means a life of self-sacrifice?	Thanks and Trust	Right action	
Tues Date: Month:	207. Ψ . . . obey the injunctions of the Ten Commandments? 208. ☺ . . . respect others' time, tastes, privacy, beliefs, opinions and feelings? [M] Who knows that I love them? How?	Discipline and discipleship	Right attitude	
Wed Date: Month:	209. Ψ . . . pray for guidance before taking action? 210. ☺ . . . remain uncomplaining about my lot? Guard my tongue? [M] Where do I fail to do those things I know I ought to do?	Prayer and Praise	Right avoidance	
Thur Date: Month:	211. Ψ . . . rest in the Lord? 212. ☺ . . . love the inner person more than the outer shell? [M] What brings me joy?	Faith and Friendship	Right attitude	
Fri Date: Month:	213. Ψ . . . follow God's injunction to "Be perfect"? 214. ☺ . . . do what I knew should be done? Work diligently, honestly? [M] When do I find myself acting inconsistently with my highest values?	Repentance and renewal	Right action	
Sat Date: Month:	215. Ψ . . . look to Jesus, his words and deeds? 216. ☺ . . . avoid complaining, blaming and passing the buck? [M] How do I feel about myself most of the time—and why?	Learning and listening	Right avoidance	
	TOTAL WEEKLY SCORE			

Sunday weekly journal:

_____

_____

_____

_____

Week 31

Training tip
Many athletes have a coach. Spiritual athletes also have a coach in the form of a spiritual counsellor. Perhaps you should review the progress you have made with a spiritual counsellor.

Words of encouragement
Let your gentleness be evident to all. The Lord is near. Philippians 4:5

Perseverance points. Tick one block every day you do the exercises

1-10%	2-20%	3-40%	4-60%	5-80%	6-100%

LOVING YOUR NEIGHBOUR
There are some people who find every excuse in the book to explain why they are NOT doing anything significant in service for their fellow-human beings. That kind of self-serving attitude runs contrary to our Lord's teachings on Christian life (refer to Matthew 5:7).

But having said that, we need to be realistic about how we serve others. It is not a good idea to let every Tom, Dick and Hilda decide your priorities. It is far better to spend time on your knees every morning (or possibly the night before) planning the day with God so that he can alert you to what needs doing for the day. Allowing God to set your priorities applies as much to those who control others as to those who have others telling them what to do.

Sometimes there will be nothing much: sometimes he really wants you to have a rest! It is possible to be so busy helping others that we have no time for Jesus himself, or for our own families or colleagues. While we are to serve God, often the way of serving him is through service to others. It is important that we keep our perspective and check all the time that we are not being trapped into the kind of busy-ness that robs us and our nearest and dearest of any meaningful spiritual life. We need to fit into God's big picture.

Having said all that, we need to be ready to help others.

Thought for the week
What most people need to learn in life is how to love people and use things instead of using people and loving things.

Love is that condition in which the happiness of another person is essential to your own. Robert A. Heinlein

WEEK 32 (& 45)

Did I . . .		Ψ	☺	TOTAL
Mon Date: Month:	217. Ψ . . . take care not to make others stumble? 218. ☺ . . . refrain from indiscretions I should have avoided? [M] Who should I see more of? Less of?	Repentance and renewal	Right avoidance	
Tues Date: Month:	219. Ψ . . . thank God for guarding and protecting me? 220. ☺ . . . avoid over-reacting when things did not go my way? [M] What habits or faults must I get rid of?	Thanks and Trust	Right avoidance	
Wed Date: Month:	221. Ψ . . . adopt a reverent bodily attitude in my prayer times? 222. ☺ . . . give alms without patronage? Forgive others? [M] Why do I worry about the future if I trust God's goodness?	Prayer and Praise	Right action	
Thur Date: Month:	223. Ψ . . . carry my Cross courageously? Anticipate and avoid evil? 224. ☺ . . . work hard to support my boss? Go the extra mile for work colleagues? [M] Where is the solution to any difficulty I face?	Discipline and discipleship	Right action	
Fri Date: Month:	225. Ψ . . . recall any words of guidance from a spiritual counsellor? 226. ☺ . . . give someone else most of the credit for positive joint actions? [M] How am I making the most of what I have been given?	Learning and listening	Right attitude	
Sat Date: Month:	227. Ψ . . . cling to God throughout the day? 228. ☺ . . . remain loving? [M] When do I NOT put my trust in God?	Faith and Friendship	Right attitude	
	TOTAL WEEKLY SCORE			

Sunday weekly journal:

_____

_____

_____

_____

Week 32

Training tip
Practice makes perfect. No one gets physically fit just by thinking about it. Neither do you get spiritually fit that way. There may be some actions you need to start doing, and some you need to stop doing.

Words of encouragement
For the LORD will vindicate his people and have compassion on his servants. Psalm 135:14

Perseverance points. Tick one block every day you do the exercises

1-10%	2-20%	3-40%	4-60%	5-80%	6-100%

SERVING OTHERS
There are those who feel guilty all the time, and are always afraid that they have not done enough. For example, they recall Jesus' injunction to "Be perfect—as your heavenly Father is perfect". They then start to think: "Shouldn't I go off and join the leprosy mission?" etc. even though they are totally unsuitable for the task. They start to worry: "Is the devil causing me to become slack, not doing enough for God?"

One man we know was quite unable to pass by anyone who seemed to need help. He spent his time picking up strangers, giving others money, blankets and clothing. He was often away from his family doing this good deed and the next. Very kind. Except he had a disabled wife who would sometimes have to sit for hours on end in the car. We could never rely on him because he was always 'out on an errand'. His household budget was a mess. His children suffered badly with his many absences and grew up not having much regard for a Lord who constantly took their father a way from them, and who caused their mother great hardship and worry.

This gathering of guilt is not a helpful, and, I would think, not an obedient thing to do. It is evident from Scripture that God does not want us to feel guilty all the time. Guilt steals our energy and prevents us from being joyfully obedient to the promptings of the Holy Spirit.

Thought for the week
Never be haughty to the humble; never be humble to the haughty. Jefferson Davis

We are all pencils in the hands of a writing God who is sending love letters to the world. Mother Theresa.

WEEK 33 (& 46)

Did I . . .		Ψ	☺	TOTAL
Mon Date: Month:	229. Ψ . . . remain alert to God speaking to me in dreams, circumstances, or through others? 230. ☺ . . . make my marriage holy? Yield when wrong? Remain loyal and loving? [M] When do I feel most fulfilled?	Learning and listening	Right action	
Tues Date: Month:	231. Ψ . . . sanctify every task, no matter how small, as an act of worship? 232. ☺ . . . put myself in the other person's shoes? Remain sensitive? [M] How do I battle my worst faults?	Prayer and Praise	Right attitude	
Wed Date: Month:	233. Ψ . . . practise abstinence, fasting, self-sacrifice, self-discipline? 234. ☺ . . . ignore petty slights, responding with love? Really desire what is best for others? [M] What must I sow in order to reap?	Discipline and discipleship	Right attitude	
Thur Date: Month:	235. Ψ . . . trust God in moments of adversity? 236. ☺ . . . delight to do God's will? Show kindness and gentleness? [M] Why do I say I love God?	Thanks and Trust	Right action	
Fri Date: Month:	237. Ψ . . . truly believe that Jesus loves me deeply? 238. ☺ . . . avoid trying to appear more learned and holy than I am? [M] Where will it all end?	Faith and Friendship	Right avoidance	
Sat Date: Month:	239. Ψ . . . guard against vanity, prejudice, procrastination, jealousy? 240. ☺ . . . avoid useless thoughts? Battle my worst faults? [M] Who are my role models in life?	Repentance and renewal	Right avoidance	
	TOTAL WEEKLY SCORE			

Sunday weekly journal:

_____

_____

_____

_____

Week 33

Training tip
To replenish their physical strength, athletes eat the right foodstuffs. The right spiritual foodstuff is the Word of God. Replenish yourself daily.

Words of encouragement
Yet I am always with you; you hold me by my right hand. You guide me with your counsel, and afterward you will take me into glory. Psalm 73: 23-24

Perseverance points. Tick one block every day you do the exercises

1-10%	2-20%	3-40%	4-60%	5-80%	6-100%

SPIRITUAL MANNERS

Mother Julian, in her wonderful little book "Revelations" speaks of "Our courteous Lord" and certainly God is most courteous when dealing with us. Revelation 3:20 tells us that he "stands at the door" of our hearts "and knocks"—waiting for our invitation to enter. He shows infinite respect and courtesy to us, and we should do no less to those around us.

There can be few people more scary (and less helpful to our spiritual growth) than the person who is so keen to help that they try to take over our lives. This can mean never leaving us alone, asking invasive questions, giving unasked-for advice, and so on. Many, many people have turned away from Christianity because of over-zealous people, desperate to make disciples—whether or not the 'disciples' were willing!

Do we really know better than others how they should live their lives? Only the very highly qualified and experienced may presume to intrude and set a new course of action. We may pray for others, show concern if they take us into their confidence, but we need to be humble and ready to acknowledge our own inadequacy. If you want to be a reformer, begin with yourself!

Spiritual manners also apply to our relationship with our heavenly Father. You worry that he does not respond to you in the way you like. Why? Do you think God does not know what he is doing? The polite and courteous thing to do is to wait on him—whether it takes a few months or a lifetime!

Thought for the week
Envy and fear cause the face to pale, and love makes it glow. Paramhansa Yogananda

Knowing is not enough, we must apply. Willing is not enough, we must do. Goethe

WEEK 34 (& 47)

Did I . . .		Ψ	☺	TOTAL
Mon Date: Month:	241. Ψ . . . strengthen my will to love God? 242. ☺ . . . avoid saying anything that discourages? Avoid inflammatory speech? [M] Where will I go when I die?	Repentance and renewal	Right avoidance	
Tues Date: Month:	243. Ψ . . . have enough faith to put my whole life in God's hands? 244. ☺ . . . love my neighbour as myself? Act with charity? [M] When am I too self-seeking or double-minded?	Faith and Friendship	Right action	
Wed Date: Month:	245. Ψ . . . make time to listen to what God wanted to say to me today? 246. ☺ . . . act in a Christian way to all? ? Reassure others? [M] What are the major obstacles I face right now?	Learning and listening	Right action	
Thur Date: Month:	247. Ψ . . . have full confidence in God? 248. ☺ . . . continue to strive for good despite rebuffs? [M] Who is the most saintly person I know?	Thanks and Trust	Right attitude	
Fri Date: Month:	249. Ψ . . . remember God in times of trial or tribulation? 250. ☺ . . . refuse to participate in any activity that was morally degrading? [M] Why am I not more whole-hearted in some of my actions?	Discipline and discipleship	Right avoidance	
Sat Date: Month:	251. Ψ . . . pray expectantly, confidently, diligently, with child-like trust? 252. ☺ . . . put the best construction on others motives and actions? [M] How else could I help God's work in the world?	Prayer and Praise	Right attitude	
	TOTAL WEEKLY SCORE			

Sunday weekly journal:

_____

_____

_____

_____

Week 34

Training tip
Remind yourself why you are doing these exercises. In the long run, your point score is unimportant. What is important is growing in spiritual maturity and strength and drawing closer to God.

Words of encouragement
What does the Scripture say? "Abraham believed God, and it was credited to him as righteousness." Romans 4:3

Perseverance points. Tick one block every day you do the exercises

1-10%	2-20%	3-40%	4-60%	5-80%	6-100%

LIVING RESPECTFULLY
Christian living entails respect for the other—maintaining complete confidentiality, not invading their privacy, allowing for their views even when they differ from ours, listening carefully, without interruption and without needing to tell our own experiences! It also entails respect for their emotions and bodies.

We help others by the way we live. If we
- keep our promises,
- listen with respect,
- apologise for mistakes,
- put a guard on our tongues,
- never bad-mouth anyone else,
- love the unloved and marginalised,
- respect the boundaries of others, and
- demonstrate loyalty,
. . . we will go a long way to witnessing to the life of God within us.

The way we react to emergencies; the way we respond to hurts and disappointments; the way we deal with relationships, with grief and with joy, will all say far more about Jesus than any words we can use. Being able to embrace differences with interest and enjoyment, being able to love in the face of resistance, mirror our Lord brightly.

We help people more by our unconscious behaviour than we can ever do in our words. Mind you, the words will be needed as well!

We need to serve others in love and sacrificial living, but we also need to be sensitive to the Holy Spirit in our own lives so that we never lose our own walk with God. To be useful to him, we need to be full of life and ready for service—not worn out and resentful.

Thought for the week
The strongest attraction to Christianity is a well-made Christian character.—Theodore Ledyard Cuyler

The greatest good you can do for another is not just to share your riches but to reveal to him his own. Benjamin Disraeli

WEEK 35 (& 48)

Did I . . .		Ψ	☺	TOTAL
Mon Date: Month:	253. Ψ . . . act with restraint and self-control with Jesus as my exemplary model? 254. ☺ . . . act as a counsellor? ? Listen carefully, always willing to share? [M] How can I do more to help my neighbour?	Discipline and discipleship	Right action	
Tues Date: Month:	255. Ψ . . . turn to the Lord for help when facing difficulties? 256. ☺ . . . help someone feel more at peace, feel good about themselves? [M] Who gives me the greatest moments of happiness in my life?	Faith and Friendship	Right attitude	
Wed Date: Month:	257. Ψ . . . accept sufferings as an opportunity for spiritual growth? 258. ☺ . . . give willingly when asked? Thank anyone who helped me? [M] When am I most often at fault?	Repentance and renewal	Right action	
Thur Date: Month:	259. Ψ . . . rely on God's liberality and generosity? 260. ☺ . . . avoid turning a blind eye in cases of moral wrong? [M] Where do I notice God at work?	Thanks and Trust	Right avoidance	
Fri Date: Month:	261. Ψ . . . pray the 'Lord's prayer' slowly and carefully? 262. ☺ . . . treat all with compassion, discretion, patience, and sincerity? [M] Why do I sometimes fail to hallow God's name?	Prayer and Praise	Right attitude	
Sat Date: Month:	263. Ψ . . . spend some time in contemplation? 264. ☺ . . . avoid sexual temptations, other thoughts or acts unworthy of God? [M] What thoughts do I need to control?	Learning and listening	Right avoidance	
	TOTAL WEEKLY SCORE			

Sunday weekly journal:

_____

_____

_____

_____

Week 35

Training tip
Self-discipline is not easy for anyone. What these exercises will help you do is to build new habits, and to help you live your Christian life, in a caring, compassionate, and self-controlled way.

Words of encouragement
Therefore, prepare your minds for action; be self-controlled; set your hope fully on the grace to be given to you when Jesus Christ is revealed. 1 Peter 1:13

Perseverance points. Tick one block every day you do the exercises

1-10%	2-20%	3-40%	4-60%	5-80%	6-100%

IS MONEY A BAD THING?

Of course not—although the excessive love of money can easily lead us astray. We start to look down on people without money as though money is the measure of our abilities, achievements and self-worth. We can buy our way out of trouble. We can sedate ourselves with expensive holidays, parties, and the so-called good things of life—forgetting what is really important, namely the glorification of God and the salvation of our souls.

Poverty is not good either. It destroys the quality of life. It creates tremendous hardship. It means we have to forgo many opportunities, for higher education and so on. Poverty deprives us of the pleasure of giving.

So what should our attitude to money be? First, we should recognize that it is God's gift to us. If we have earned it though our talents, who has given us those talents? If we are heirs to a large fortune, God's hand is also at work there. Second, we should recognize that money is opportunity—an opportunity to share and give, an opportunity to help the disadvantaged, an opportunity to glorify God in a way that will not be open to people without money.

To grow in the spiritual life, consider the pathway of voluntary simplicity in which we spend only what we have to and don't waste. We should learn to manage and control our money well just as we nurture and look after any other talents we may have been given. But we should not let money rule our lives.

Thought for the week
Live simply so that others may simply live. Mahatma Gandhi

When you don't know what you want, you end up wanting a lot more than you need. Floyd Maxwell

WEEK 36 (& 49)

Did I . . .		Ψ	☺	TOTAL
Mon Date: Month:	265. Ψ . . . remain still and silent before God before starting to pray? 266. ☺ . . . refuse to justify an action I should not have done? [M] Why do I do it?	Prayer and Praise	Right avoidance	
Tues Date: Month:	267. Ψ . . . study systematically rather than at random? 268. ☺ . . . use my gifts for the good of others? Do what I ought to do? [M] How can I become more serene and tranquil?	Learning and listening	Right attitude	
Wed Date: Month:	269. Ψ . . . have faith that despite my sins I was not condemned? 270. ☺ . . . put my religious or beliefs into practice? [M Where does my real passion lie?	Faith and Friendship	Right attitude	
Thur Date: Month:	271. Ψ . . . . thank God for any good I may have done? 272. ☺ . . . do a good deed? Go the extra mile to help someone? [M] When does God seem most real in my life?	Thanks and Trust	Right action	
Fri Date: Month:	273. Ψ . . . scrupulously avoid what is forbidden or dangerous? 274. ☺ . . . give a gift or compliment to someone? Point out strengths? [M] Who has influenced me most in my spiritual life?	Repentance and renewal	Right action	
Sat Date: Month:	275. Ψ . . . sacrifice my desires by putting God's will first? 276. ☺ . . . avoid miserliness, unwholesome curiosity? Refrain from resenting or envying others? [M] What mistakes do I find myself repeating?	Discipline and discipleship	Right avoidance	
	TOTAL WEEKLY SCORE			

Sunday weekly journal:

_____

_____

_____

_____

Week 36

Training tip
In any training programme, there are times when you can over-strain. Or you may face headwinds. Or perhaps you are disappointed with your progress. Simply do the best you can each day. That's all there is to it.

Words of encouragement
Blessed are they whose ways are blameless, who walk according to the law of the LORD. Psalm 119:1

Perseverance points. Tick one block every day you do the exercises

1-10%	2-20%	3-40%	4-60%	5-80%	6-100%

TITHING
"The earth is the LORD'S, and everything in it." (Psalm 24:1) What we call our own is only entrusted to us so that we can use it for God and his people. After all, if God wishes to provide money for a project, usually it will come through someone's bank account. We work carefully with what we have so that we will have enough when he asks us to pass it on. We can then freely give it, for the same God who is providing for the other, will also provide for us.

You can see the happy implications. I need never panic about my financial situation as long as I act according to God's plan. The rule of tithing is this: 10% of everything we get goes straight out to God's work. Usually this means that we give it to our Church, although having a small fund for emergency requests is also okay.

People sometimes ask, "Is it 10% before tax or after?" "Shouldn't I first pay my expenses and then give away?" Sensible questions. The answer, however, is NO. As you give your 10% *off the top, before anything else is paid*, God sees to it that what you have left is enough, and usually more than enough. We don't always have to FEEL faith—we can just act it out. Tithing is a perfect example of this. Read Malachi 3 verse 10 and take it to heart. (In fact, read the whole chapter.) This may be the turning point in your financial security!

Thought for the week
It is always better to give than to receive. Be a river, not a swamp.

At present we have a society based on having and owning; we need a society based around being and giving. Mike Scott

WEEK 37 (& 50)

Did I . . .		Ψ	☺	TOTAL
Mon Date: Month:	277. Ψ . . . trust God's word in the Bible? 278. ☺ . . . persevere in doing good to all? Turn the other cheek? [M] Who needs more of my love and affection and caring?	Thanks and Trust	Right attitude	
Tues Date: Month:	279. Ψ . . . strive to know and do God's will? 280. ☺ . . . help someone? Comfort? Nurture? Assist? Make a sacrifice? [M] Why do I not trust more in God and his loving kindness and strength?	Repentance and renewal	Right action	
Wed Date: Month:	281. Ψ . . . take great comfort from the love of God? 282. ☺ . . . make people sincerely feel I had their interests at heart? [M] How can I live more simply?	Faith and Friendship	Right attitude	
Thur Date: Month:	283. Ψ . . . pray with positive expectations of guidance from the Holy Spirit? 284. ☺ . . . relentlessly ght my bad tendencies? Avoid all evil thoughts? [M] What do I do when I get stressed?	Prayer and Praise	Right avoidance	
Fri Date: Month:	285. Ψ . . . behave as I believe God wanted me to? 286. ☺ . . . avoid taking pleasure in others misfortunes? [M] When do I feel being a Christian is most worthwhile?	Discipline and discipleship	Right avoidance	
Sat Date: Month:	287. Ψ . . . increase my knowledge of God in any way? 288. ☺ . . . surprise someone with a gift of kindness? [M] Where do I want to spend the rest of my life?	Learning and listening	Right action	
	TOTAL WEEKLY SCORE			

Sunday weekly journal:

_____

_____

_____

_____

Week 37

Training tip
You may find yourself thinking, "I could have done so much better today." That's a sign of progress. When we truly realise the unutterable holiness of God, we will always fall short.

Words of encouragement
And God is able to make all grace abound to you, so that in all things at all times, having all that you need, you will abound in every good work. 2 Corinthians 9:8

Perseverance points. Tick one block every day you do the exercises

1-10%	2-20%	3-40%	4-60%	5-80%	6-100%

TEMPTATION

Don't think for a moment that having Jesus as Lord of your life will mean an end to temptation and difficulties. Jesus told his disciples, "In the world you will have trouble. But take heart! I have overcome the world". (John 16:33) Things may still go terribly wrong, and we may still be tempted to sin, perhaps even more fiercely than before.

Satan will roll out everything he has got to draw those he can't destroy, into sin again. It certainly seems that the closer you get to God, the sharper the temptations become. It stands to reason—the more you are relying on God, the more lost you are to Satan and the harder he will try to win you back.

Satan has another strategy up his sleeve. He tempts you to think little sins are "not too bad". Thus we have greed masquerading as a healthy appetite, physical pride and vanity pretending to be merely the quest for the perfect body, and "being realistic" too often used as an excuse for complacency and indifference. We give in to gossip and the "fellowship of disparagement". We pass the buck. All these, some say, are perfectly normal!

Many people find that immediately after an event or experience that has lifted them into a high spiritual place, where they are deeply blessed, the wheels fall off and everything goes wrong. I have learnt to view this as a kind of confirmation that the experience I have just had is real and must be very right for Satan to get so panicky!

Thought for the week
Be not simply good; be good for something. Henry David Thoreau (1817-1862)

God seeks comrades and claims love,
The Devil seeks slaves and claims obedience.
Rabindranath Tagore

WEEK 38 (& 51)

Did I . . .		Ψ	☺	**TOTAL**
Mon Date: Month:	289. Ψ . . . treat my body as a holy temple? Fight the good fight? 290. ☺ . . . keep my promises and fulfil all my obligations? [M] What would make for an ideal family life?	Discipline and discipleship	Right attitude	
Tues Date: Month:	291. Ψ . . . thank God for sustenance of soul and body? 292. ☺ . . . help others not to stumble? Forgo an advantage? [M] Why do I let myself slip back from my high standards?	Thanks and Trust	Right attitude	
Wed Date: Month:	293. Ψ . . . rejoice in the Lord, enjoying my prayer time with Him? 294. ☺ . . . bless any house/workplace I entered? Pray for someone? [M] Where is the greatest need that I can do something about?	Prayer and Praise	Right action	
Thur Date: Month:	295. Ψ . . . memorise/recall any Bible passages? 296. ☺ . . . give a donation? Make amends for wrongdoing? [M] How would I live the perfect Christian life?	Learning and listening	Right action	
Fri Date: Month:	297. Ψ . . . address my predominant fault by cultivating the opposite virtue? 298. ☺ . . . keep any negative, critical or sad thoughts to myself? [M] Who needs help where I can make a difference?	Repentance and renewal	Right avoidance	
Sat Date: Month:	299. Ψ . . . maintain my faith despite problems? 300. ☺ . . . repress impure thoughts? Avoid hardness of heart or resentment? [M] When am I at my best? Worst?	Faith and Friendship	Right avoidance	
	TOTAL WEEKLY SCORE			

Sunday weekly journal:

_____

_____

_____

_____

Week 38

Training tip
"Right effort" is in a sense, effortless. Those who are well trained in any sport find it easier to perform well. When you find yourself doing the right act almost without thinking about it, this is real progress.

Words of encouragement
Surely goodness and love will follow me all the days of my life, and I will dwell in the house of the LORD forever. Psalm 23:6

Perseverance points. Tick one block every day you do the exercises

1-10%	2-20%	3-40%	4-60%	5-80%	6-100%

DOES GOD TEST US?

I often hear people saying, "God sends us temptation to test our faith." I am not sure that he needs to do that. He knows our faith, how strong or delicate it is. After all, our faith is a gift from him, so he hardly needs to test it out to find out if it is working or not.

But in another sense, I believe that he does test us. That is, the kind of testing that helps us to grow and learn spiritually. In the same way as practice strengthens skill, so we develop our skills and holy habits in the face of temptation. I learn to ride a bike by resisting the pull of falling off and my balance gets better and better as I overcome this pull time and again, both when the going is smooth and when the going is rough. I know what to do when conditions are difficult. In a similar way, the existence of the pull of sin, when it is overcome, strengthens me in my spiritual 'balance'.

God certainly allows Satan to tempt us, to try to dislodge our peace, to push us almost to the edge. Fear not! God stands with us and offers his arm in the midst of the attack, and he has promised that "he will not let you be tempted beyond what you can bear" (1 Corinthians 10:13). And each time we stand firm in his strength, we become a little stronger, a bit spiritually smarter, and closer to the glory of his likeness in our lives.

Thought for the week
I see more and more that what Jesus Christ wants of you is that you abandon yourself without reserve to His will and His love. Dom Marmion

Truth hurts. Not the searching after, the running from. John Eyberg

WEEK 39 (& 52)

Did I . . .		Ψ	☺	TOTAL
Mon Date: Month:	301 Ψ . . . stick to the straight and narrow? Avoid worldly ambition? 302 ☺ . . . avoid devious behaviour, covetousness? Trying to dominate? [M] When am I inclined to be judgemental or self-righteous?	Repentance and renewal	Right avoidance	
Tues Date: Month:	303 Ψ . . . give thanks for strength in time of trials? 304 ☺ . . . act with gentleness? Share privileges? [M] Where do I fall down in my spiritual life?	Thanks and Trust	Right attitude	
Wed Date: Month:	305 Ψ . . . seek guidance through books or others to help me understand God's word? 306 ☺ . . . refuse to entertain false beliefs? Avoid upsetting others? [M] Who is the best judge of my character and ability?	Learning and listening	Right avoidance	
Thur Date: Month:	307 Ψ . . . desire to make sacrifices for God? 308 ☺ . . . pray for others when I was unable to help? [M] What behaviours do I need to cultivate?	Discipline and discipleship	Right action	
Fri Date: Month:	309 Ψ . . . allow silences in my prayers waiting to hear God's voice? 310 ☺ . . . relieve others of worry, pain, distress, loss or despair? [M] How often do I read the Bible?	Prayer and Praise	Right action	
Sat Date: Month:	311 Ψ . . . hold firm to my belief that God cares about me? 312 ☺ . . . sacrifice my comfort for others? [M] Why am I certain that God is love?	Faith and Friendship	Right attitude	
	TOTAL WEEKLY SCORE			

Sunday weekly journal:

_____

_____

_____

_____

Week 39

Training tip

The greatest stumbling block in making progress in the spiritual life is pride. By ourselves we can do nothing. Always remind yourself that it is God working through you that enables you to grow.

Words of encouragement

For with you is the fountain of life; in your light we see light. Psalm 36:9

Perseverance points. Tick one block every day you do the exercises

1-10%	2-20%	3-40%	4-60%	5-80%	6-100%

TEMPTATION FROM WITHIN

The worst kind of temptation usually doesn't come from friends or events—outside of us. The most insidious temptations come through our own thoughts and emotions—from within.

I often find it difficult to pray, not because there is no time but because I just don't feel like it. I have more difficulty controlling my unruly nature than dealing with interruptions and time pressures. Because I find it hard to control my feelings or pull myself out of a mood, it can be really hard settling down to pray, until I remember who it is that I am not wanting to spend time with. My lover! The one whose presence I long to have burst in on me like the bright rays of the early morning sun, and whose love I crave to feel filling every fibre of my being. Is that stupid or what?

Can you see that this unwillingness to spend time with him is not really from me, but is the subtle temptation that Satan feeds into my mind so that I will pay attention to it? And it turns on my forgetting the truth about God and his amazing love and grace and kindness and longing for me to come into his presence. If you face this problem, deal with it by consciously bringing your mind to dwell on this truth as you pray.

Whatever the temptation it is that you face—pride, envy, gluttony, sloth,—remember that you are not your own. You were bought at a great price. God fights your temptation right there at your side.

Thought for the week

The devil appeared to St Bridget, and she asked him: "What is your name?"
"Coldness itself." Abbé Huvelin

Motto of a Bible-reading family: A chapter a day keeps the devil away.

WEEK 40 (& 27)

Did I . . .		Ψ	☺	TOTAL
Mon Date: Month:	157. Ψ . . . behave in a way pleasing to him? Rely on God completely? 158. ☺ . . . create contentment rather than discontent? Share a smile? [M] When do I feel closest to God?	Repentance and renewal	Right attitude	
Tues Date: Month:	159. Ψ . . . praise God in all His majesty? 160 ☺ . . . give of my time, money, energy or talent to help others? [M] Why do I sometimes feel depressed? What should I do about it?	Prayer and Praise	Right action	
Wed Date: Month:	161. Ψ . . . do what Jesus would have me to do—despite difficulties? 162. ☺ . . . refrain from childishness, recklessness? Avoid prejudice? [M] How do I show I love God?	Discipline and discipleship	Right avoidance	
Thur Date: Month:	163. Ψ . . . have faith in God's holy laws? 164. ☺ . . . avoid becoming over-anxious? Avoid behaving rashly? [M] Where are opportunities for me to do good?	Faith and Friendship	Right avoidance	
Fri Date: Month:	165. Ψ . . . ask for divine inspiration before starting to study God's word? 166. ☺ . . . exercise compassion expecting nothing in return? [M] What energises me?	Learning and listening	Right attitude	
Sat Date: Month:	167. Ψ . . . act as a trusty steward in the position that God placed me? 168. ☺ . . . say something to make people feel that they mattered? Empathize? [M] Who is my neighbour?	Thanks and Trust	Right action	
	TOTAL WEEKLY SCORE			

Sunday weekly journal:

_____

_____

_____

_____

Week 40

Training tip
You are about to repeat the third quarter's questions again. Many runners use a heart rate monitor to measure their heart rate. The comparative scorecards give you a chance to perform even better than last time.

Words of encouragement
Great peace have they who love your law, And nothing can make them stumble. Psalm 119:165

Perseverance points. Tick one block every day you do the exercises

1-10%	2-20%	3-40%	4-60%	5-80%	6-100%

UNWILLING HOLINESS
It's terribly easy to put off being righteous and holy. Often we are more inclined to take the line of least resistance, to go with the prompting of our lower nature rather than to hold out for what we know is good and right and lasting. We often forget how vital the 'imitation of Christ' is!

Remember the story of the man who died. He was greeted on the other side by St Peter who asked him whether he would prefer to go to heaven or hell. He asked to have a look first so that he could make an informed decision. He was shown heaven first, with people going around with happy faces, quietly and lovingly living. He was impressed. Then he looked into hell and saw everyone having a wild party—eating, drinking, flirting, dancing,—and having a ball. That looked like his sort of thing. He chose hell.

Immediately he was whisked off into the darkness and torture of a most awful kind. As he shrieked in agony he asked Satan what had become of the hell he had seen. Satan's reply was, 'Oh that! That's just our marketing package!"

In physical training, few people really like getting up in the cold of dawn and going to the gym. Yet they do so because they want results. The result we long for is to hear God say, "Well done, good and faithful servant'. (Matthew 25:21) To hear him say that makes everything worthwhile.

Thought for the week
The Beauty of life is to Give
The Joy of life is to Love.
William Arthur Ward

Sanctity does not consist merely in doing the will of God. It consists in willing the will of God. For sanctity is in union with God . . . Thomas Merton

WEEK 41 (& 28)

Did I . . .		Ψ	☺	TOTAL
Mon Date: Month:	169. Ψ . . . read the Bible or other religious texts prayerfully, carefully and remain open to the truth? 170. ☺ . . . avoid being self-righteous? Avoid being presumptuous and swollen-headed? [M] Where is God?	Learning and listening	Right Avoidance	
Tues Date: Month:	171. Ψ . . . strive for purity of heart? Avoid inordinate desires? 172. ☺ . . . give alms, a gift, or courage to others? Cheer anyone up? [M] When am I a good listener?	Repentance and renewal	Right action	
Wed Date: Month:	173. Ψ . . . examine the causes of, or reasons for, any doubts? 174. ☺ . . . try to understand others' needs, tastes, frustrations, hopes? Reach out? [M] Why do I not have a vision for my life? (if I don't)	Faith and Friendship	Right attitude	
Thur Date: Month:	175. Ψ . . . say 'flash prayers' during the day for others? 176. ☺ . . . behave with hospitality? Help the underprivileged? [M] How do I practice self-denial?	Prayer and Praise	Right action	
Fri Date: Month:	177. Ψ . . . do what God wanted, acting diligently at all times? 178. ☺ . . . give more than would be expected from common decency? [M] Who do I dislike most—and why?	Discipline and discipleship	Right attitude	
Sat Date: Month:	179. Ψ . . . conclude my prayers with thanks? 180. ☺ . . . avoid comparisons with another? Refrain from being petty? [M] What are my best and worst qualities?	Thanks and Trust	Right avoidance	
	TOTAL WEEKLY SCORE			

Sunday weekly journal:

_____

_____

_____

_____

Week 41

Training tip
There is an ancient proverb that says, "Truthfulness is the holy person's root". We delude ourselves seriously when we over-value our own contribution. But don't 'run yourself down' either. Simply forge ahead!

Words of encouragement
When my spirit grows faint within me, it is you who know my way. Psalm 142:3

Perseverance points. Tick one block every day you do the exercises

1-10%	2-20%	3-40%	4-60%	5-80%	6-100%

PRACTISING RECEIVING GOD'S LOVE

A single parent struggling to house and feed her children on a small salary received an anonymous letter in the postbox. "An amount of $1 000 has been paid into an account for you at—(the local supermarket). Please buy whatever you want." She could not think where it came from and was too afraid to risk going to the shop in case it was a hoax. So she avoided that shop and went right on struggling.

This is a terribly sad story. The woman in question could not believe that she was worthy of this sort of support from someone she didn't even know, so she did not take up the offer. She doubted the truth of the message and refused the loving gift because she felt unworthy. Of course, we know that 'worthy' and 'gift' are not connected. A gift is given irrespective of worth.

With God, we already know that we are unworthy. So the idea of being worthy of God's grace is silly. If we refuse to believe that he loves us, if we refuse to act as if we are God's darlings, we are just like that mother.

Trust him. Believe that his promises are true. Live as one who is loved by God. The more you do it, the more you will know it. Just *act as if* he loves you and do the next thing. If that mother had *acted as if,* she would have gone to the supermarket and shopped.

Thought for the week
The shell must break before the bird can fly. Alfred, Lord Tennyson.

He that gives should never remember, he that receives should never forget. Talmud

WEEK 42 (& 29)

Did I . . .		Ψ	☺	TOTAL
Mon Date: Month:	181. Ψ . . . pray meaningful and not empty words? 182. ☺ . . . behave sensitively? Make sure I did not cause offence? [M] How can I be of more service to others?	Prayer and Praise	Right attitude	
Tues Date: Month:	183. Ψ . . . meditate on God's precepts? 184. ☺ . . . renounce inordinate self-love? Renounce my own will? [M] Where do I do my best work?	Learning and listening	Right avoidance	
Wed Date: Month:	185. Ψ . . . trust God to answer my prayers? 186. ☺ . . . pay debts promptly? Thank? Treat others generously? [M] When am I most truly 'myself'?	Thanks and Trust	Right action	
Thur Date: Month:	187. Ψ . . . strive mightily to eradicate faults as well as ask for God's help? 188. ☺ . . . avoid letting others get me down through negative talk? [M] Who dislikes me—and why?	Repentance and renewal	Right avoidance	
Fri Date: Month:	189. Ψ . . . believe that God wants to be my friend? 190. ☺ . . . give, do or say something unexpectedly nice for someone? [M] What is it I really love and why?	Faith and Friendship	Right action	
Sat Date: Month:	191. Ψ . . . endure sufferings or difficulties with patience? 192. ☺ . . . strive to be a blessing to others? ? Listen with care rather than foster my own opinion on others? [M] Why am I doing these exercises?	Discipline and discipleship	Right attitude	
	TOTAL WEEKLY SCORE			

Sunday weekly journal:

_____

_____

_____

_____

Week 42

Training tip

Each day has enough troubles of its own. Don't worry about the past. Don't worry about the future. Take each day as it comes. God wants your happiness.

Words of encouragement

If a man remains in me and I in him, he will bear much fruit; apart from me you can do nothing. John 15:5

Perseverance points. Tick one block every day you do the exercises

1-10%	2-20%	3-40%	4-60%	5-80%	6-100%

GETTING DAILY GUIDANCE

Start every day with a period of quiet with God. That means not talking, not doing anything, except filling your mind with him and resting in him. The process is a bit like sitting silently in a room with someone you love, or a mother watching her baby sleep peacefully. Simply enjoy the moment.

Have your notebook or your diary handy and write down the things that come to mind as you think about the day. Do exactly what God directs in this morning prayer time—sometimes certain things come into sharp focus: do them as a priority. Other planned activities may become clearly less important, and you may even realise that some would be a mistake as God shows you implications you had not seen before.

Doing what needs to be done—and doing it well—is a good way of serving God in the everyday life—even cleaning the sink!

Throughout your day, remember God is with you. When you face a crisis or problem, send him a 'flash prayer' and say, "Jesus, please help." But even if your day runs smoothly, stay alert to God's presence. One person we know sets his alarm on his wristwatch to go off at hourly intervals as a reminder to say "Thanks God."

Don't rush off after great ideas unless God confirms them for you. If you are not sure, check with a spiritual friend or with your director. God rarely inspires only one person. Remember how in Acts, St Luke says, "It seemed good to the Holy Spirit *and to us.*"

Thought for the week

Each one should remain in the situation which he was in when God called him. 1 Corinthians 7:20

There is a voice within, if only we would listen to it, that tells us so certainly when to go forth into the unknown. Elizabeth Kubler-Ross

WEEK 43 (& 30)

Did I . . .		Ψ	☺	TOTAL
Mon Date: Month:	193. Ψ . . . have faith in God's goodness rather than material wealth? 194. ☺ . . . let my Christian conviction shine forth? Forgive and forget? [M] Where do I find peace?	Faith and Friendship	Right attitude	
Tues Date: Month:	195. Ψ . . . say grace before meals? Ask blessings for others? 196. ☺ . . . avoid self-indulgence? Gluttony? Wayward behaviour? [M] What Christian attributes do I lack?	Prayer and Praise	Right avoidance	
Wed Date: Month:	197. Ψ . . . practise detachment from things? 198. ☺ . . . refuse to cover up blind spots in my moral and spiritual life? [M] Who is a source of temptation for me?	Repentance and renewal	Right avoidance	
Thur Date: Month:	199. Ψ . . . stick to my Bible reading plan? 200. ☺ . . . say kindly words? Share a smile? Congratulate? Make amends? [M] When do I feel most compassionate?	Learning and listening	Right action	
Fri Date: Month:	201. Ψ . . . give thanks for all things? Rely on Him completely? 202. ☺ . . . listen with care? Speak truthfully? Refrain from anger or bearing grudges? [M] How do I prevent stress, negativity or despondency?	Thanks and Trust	Right attitude	
Sat Date: Month:	203. Ψ . . . purge bad dispositions? Act in the right way from the right motives? 204. ☺ . . . treat all with kindness? Stand up for the faith? Say a good word? [M] Why do I pray for peace when the world is continually at war?	Discipline and discipleship	Right action	
	TOTAL WEEKLY SCORE			

Sunday weekly journal:

_____

_____

_____

_____

Week 43

Training tip
The best athletes run with a relaxed style. Tension is rarely good. These ten minutes you spend before God should be times of relaxed concentration. Are you relaxed?

Words of encouragement
The Spirit of God has made me, the breath of the Almighty gives me life. Job 33:4

Perseverance points. Tick one block every day you do the exercises

1-10%	2-20%	3-40%	4-60%	5-80%	6-100%

CHECKING OUT A COURSE OF ACTION
"How can I know when it is God speaking?" is a question often asked.

Firstly, we get to recognise God's voice in the same way that we get to recognise the voices of our family and friends—familiarity. The more time we spend with him, the better we learn to know him. There is no short cut to knowing God and recognising his voice. This is why it is so very important to spend time reading the scriptures as well as praying (and listening in prayer!) every day.

Secondly, we are encouraged to check out with other Christians what we believe God is saying. This is one of the reasons we need to be in a fellowship group where we get to know each other on a deep level and are able to trust each other with confidences.

One way of getting guidance is discussing what the situation is, mentioning the alternatives you have identified, listening to other suggestions, then going to prayer, asking the Holy Spirit to guide you. Spend time in silence together, allowing your thoughts to range over what you have discussed, until something begins to stand out. It may be an idea, a question, a clear sense of direction, or nothing at all. Then each share what has become clear to you, being totally honest. There will usually be a degree of consensus as to what God is saying.

Be wary of 'guidance' that comes to you only. It may well be your own desires speaking.

Thought for the week
Use the talents you possess, for the woods would be a very silent place if no birds sang except the best. Henry Van Dyke

Man discovers his own wealth when God comes to ask gifts of him. Rabindranath Tagore

WEEK 44 (& 31)

Did I . . .		Ψ	☺	TOTAL
Mon Date: Month:	205. Ψ . . . trust God sufficiently to avoid anxiety? 206. ☺ . . . listen patiently? Give my full attention to someone with a problem? [M] Why serve God if it means a life of self-sacrifice?	Thanks and Trust	Right action	
Tues Date: Month:	207. Ψ . . . obey the injunctions of the Ten Commandments? 208. ☺ . . . respect others' time, tastes, privacy, beliefs, opinions and feelings? [M] Who knows that I love them? How?	Discipline and discipleship	Right attitude	
Wed Date: Month:	209. Ψ . . . pray for guidance before taking action? 210. ☺ . . . remain uncomplaining about my lot? Guard my tongue? [M] Where do I fail to do those things I know I ought to do?	Prayer and Praise	Right avoidance	
Thur Date: Month:	211. Ψ . . . rest in the Lord? 212. ☺ . . . love the inner person more than the outer shell? [M] What brings me joy?	Faith and Friendship	Right attitude	
Fri Date: Month:	213. Ψ . . . follow God's injunction to "Be perfect"? 214. ☺ . . . do what I knew should be done? Work diligently, honestly? [M] When do I find myself acting inconsistently with my highest values?	Repentance and renewal	Right action	
Sat Date: Month:	215. Ψ . . . look to Jesus, his words and deeds? 216. ☺ . . . avoid complaining, blaming and passing the buck? [M] How do I feel about myself most of the time—and why?	Learning and listening	Right avoidance	
	TOTAL WEEKLY SCORE			

Sunday weekly journal:

_____

_____

_____

_____

Week 44

Training tip
All of us need to learn to run towards the good, run away from evil. Don't dally along the way.

Words of encouragement
For the LORD God is a sun and shield; the LORD bestows favor and honor; no good thing does he withhold from those whose walk is blameless. Psalm 84:11

Perseverance points. Tick one block every day you do the exercises

1-10%	2-20%	3-40%	4-60%	5-80%	6-100%

A RULE OF LIFE.
It is a very good idea to write down on a piece of paper 'A rule of life' and commit yourself to this. Your 'rule of life', which will be personal to you, is your own 'set of commandments' about the standards you will uphold in daily life.

Your 'rule of life' should be a series of very simple statements perhaps one or two sentences long. Review each year modifying it, if necessary, under the guidance of the Holy Spirit.

Most 'rules' have certain headings:
1. Holy Eucharist: A commitment as to how often you will attend.
2. Penitence and Confession: Usually before a priest. Perhaps quarterly.
3. Personal prayer: How often? When? For how long?
4. Self-denial: Fasting on Friday? Moderating your intake of certain types of food?
5. Retreat: It is a good idea at least once a year to take out a few days to be alone with God. While you could do this in your own home, it is better to do this at a Retreat Centre.
6. Study: Primarily this will relate to the word of God, but it may also refer to other useful subjects. We grow or dwindle in our entirety.
7. Simplicity: Our lives and homes are inclined to become full of clutter. Action?
8. Work and service: Ethical standards? Charitable activities you will embark on?
9. Obedience: Perhaps there is something you need to do here.
10. Tithing of talent, time, and treasury: What are you going to give back to God?

Thought for the week
God grant me
Serenity to accept the things I cannot change,
Courage to change the things I can,
And wisdom to know the difference.
—*Prayer of Alcoholics Anonymous*

WEEK 45 (& 32)

Did I . . .		Ψ	☺	TOTAL
Mon Date: Month:	217. Ψ . . . take care not to make others stumble? 218. ☺ . . . refrain from indiscretions I should have avoided? [M] Who should I see more of? Less of?	Repentance and renewal	Right avoidance	
Tues Date: Month:	219. Ψ . . . thank God for guarding and protecting me? 220. ☺ . . . avoid over-reacting when things did not go my way? [M] What habits or faults must I get rid of?	Thanks and Trust	Right avoidance	
Wed Date: Month:	221. Ψ . . . adopt a reverent bodily attitude in my prayer times? 222. ☺ . . . give alms without patronage? Forgive others? [M] Why do I worry about the future if I trust God's goodness?	Prayer and Praise	Right action	
Thur Date: Month:	223. Ψ . . . carry my Cross courageously? Anticipate and avoid evil? 224. ☺ . . . work hard to support my boss? Go the extra mile for work colleagues? [M] Where is the solution to any difficulty I face?	Discipline and discipleship	Right action	
Fri Date: Month:	225. Ψ . . . recall any words of guidance from a spiritual counsellor? 226. ☺ . . . give someone else most of the credit for positive joint actions? [M] How am I making the most of what I have been given?	Learning and listening	Right attitude	
Sat Date: Month:	227. Ψ . . . cling to God throughout the day? 228. ☺ . . . remain loving? [M] When do I NOT put my trust in God?	Faith and Friendship	Right attitude	
	TOTAL WEEKLY SCORE			

Sunday weekly journal:

_____

_____

_____

_____

Week 45

Training tip
Sunday is a day of rest. Review the introductory pages to see one technique for using the comments you can put down here.

Words of encouragement
But you, O Lord, are a compassionate and gracious God, slow to anger, abounding in love and faithfulness. Psalm 86:15

Perseverance points. Tick one block every day you do the exercises

1-10%	2-20%	3-40%	4-60%	5-80%	6-100%

TURNING THE SOUL TO GOD
Growing spiritually fit is a lifetime journey. As you advance, God will guide you in his own special way. Yet there are some factors that seem to apply to all the spiritual giants. (Beware of spiritual pride!)

There is a need for deep-seated convictions about God and his word. You really do need to work these through. For example, in the Sermon on the Mount, Jesus made some very challenging statements. Are they true for you? What do they mean? An excellent book here to read is William Barclay's book called 'The Beatitudes'.

Then you will come to realize that the truly holy life is the sacrificial life—putting God and others first, foregoing certain pleasures for the greater good. This can be hugely challenging and there is nothing worse than a grumpy 'duty bound' Christian reluctantly 'giving his all' (and usually expecting to be praised for this!)

Humility is the hallmark of the holy person. Not a 'false humility' which says 'I am completely without talent and ability' but real humility in which you realize how everything you have is God's gift for your use and recognize, using God's standards, that there are so many others who are probably better than you.

Control of the passions requires constant attention. Here, sensible advice would be to attack your predominant fault and to work on this diligently before moving on to the next problem.

In summary, the challenge is self-renunciation, training the will so that base instincts have no appeal, self-discipline, and above all, turning the soul to God.

Thought for the week
Be careful what you set your heart on for it will surely be yours. Emerson

I sought my soul but my soul I could not see.
I sought my God but my God eluded me.
I sought my brother—and I found all three.
—Prayer printed in London Church News, May 1908.

WEEK 46 (& 33)

Did I . . .		Ψ	☺	**TOTAL**
Mon Date: Month:	229. Ψ . . . remain alert to God speaking to me in dreams, circumstances, or through others? 230. ☺ . . . make my marriage holy? Yield when wrong? Remain loyal and loving? [M] When do I feel most fulfilled?	Learning and listening	Right action	
Tues Date: Month:	231. Ψ . . . sanctify every task, no matter how small, as an act of worship? 232. ☺ . . . put myself in the other person's shoes? Remain sensitive? [M] How do I battle my worst faults?	Prayer and Praise	Right attitude	
Wed Date: Month:	233. Ψ . . . practise abstinence, fasting, self-sacrifice, self-discipline? 234. ☺ . . . ignore petty slights, responding with love? Really desire what is best for others? [M] What must I sow in order to reap?	Discipline and discipleship	Right attitude	
Thur Date: Month:	235. Ψ . . . trust God in moments of adversity? 236. ☺ . . . delight to do God's will? Show kindness and gentleness? [M] Why do I say I love God?	Thanks and Trust	Right action	
Fri Date: Month:	237. Ψ . . . truly believe that Jesus loves me deeply? 238. ☺ . . . avoid trying to appear more learned and holy than I am? [M] Where will it all end?	Faith and Friendship	Right avoidance	
Sat Date: Month:	239. Ψ . . . guard against vanity, prejudice, procrastination, jealousy? 240. ☺ . . . avoid useless thoughts? Battle my worst faults? [M] Who are my role models in life?	Repentance and renewal	Right avoidance	
	TOTAL WEEKLY SCORE			

Sunday weekly journal:

_____

_____

_____

_____

Week 46

Training tip
Are you examining your scores? Are there any areas that need working on?

Words of encouragement
The Lord is righteous in all his ways and loving toward all he has made. The Lord is near to all who call on him, to all who call on him in truth. Psalm 145:17-18.

Perseverance points. Tick one block every day you do the exercises

1-10%	2-20%	3-40%	4-60%	5-80%	6-100%

THE NEED FOR A MODEL

It is really helpful to have a role model in life. While books are helpful, such as the bibliographies of the saints, try to find someone in your community or church you really look up to. What does he or she say, think or do? For example, have you noticed that there are some people who never say anything bad about anyone (no matter how much it might seem to be deserved!)? Or perhaps you know of someone who always says a kind word or is enormously sensitive to others and their needs.

Of course, in Jesus, we have our perfect model. We should all strive to live a divine life. What were the special qualities about Jesus that you should try to emulate? There are many, but here are a few:
—the holiness of his actions, his exemplary prayer life, delicate sensibilities,
—compassion, humility, gentleness, pure motives, heroic courage,
—purity of intention, fervour, generosity, determination and constancy,
—utter self-effacement, horror of sin, complete obedience to his Father,
—zeal in public life, wisdom and knowledge of Scripture.

And much more. He continually gave thanks to his Father, fought temptations, endured hunger and fatigue without complaint, remained calm under pressure, was unswayed by successes and reverses, and loved and loved and loved.

We need to not simply know *about* Jesus, we need to know Him. "I am the vine, you are the branches," he said. We draw our life from Him.

Thought for the week
Christ: the life of the soul.—Book title

Jesu, my Lord, I thee adore,
O make me love thee more and more.—English hymn

WEEK 47 (& 34)

Did I . . .		Ψ	☺	TOTAL
Mon Date: Month:	241. Ψ . . . strengthen my will to love God? 242. ☺ . . . avoid saying anything that discourages? Avoid inflammatory speech? [M] Where will I go when I die?	Repentance and renewal	Right avoidance	
Tues Date: Month:	243. Ψ . . . have enough faith to put my whole life in God's hands? 244. ☺ . . . love my neighbour as myself? Act with charity? [M] When am I too self-seeking or double-minded?	Faith and Friendship	Right action	
Wed Date: Month:	245. Ψ . . . make time to listen to what God wanted to say to me today? 246. ☺ . . . act in a Christian way to all? ? Reassure others? [M] What are the major obstacles I face right now?	Learning and listening	Right action	
Thur Date: Month:	247. Ψ . . . have full confidence in God? 248. ☺ . . . continue to strive for good despite rebuffs? [M] Who is the most saintly person I know?	Thanks and Trust	Right attitude	
Fri Date: Month:	249. Ψ . . . remember God in times of trial or tribulation? 250. ☺ . . . refuse to participate in any activity that was morally degrading? [M] Why am I not more whole-hearted in some of my actions?	Discipline and discipleship	Right avoidance	
Sat Date: Month:	251. Ψ . . . pray expectantly, confidently, diligently, with child-like trust? 252. ☺ . . . put the best construction on others motives and actions? [M] How else could I help God's work in the world?	Prayer and Praise	Right attitude	
	TOTAL WEEKLY SCORE			

Sunday weekly journal:

_____

_____

_____

_____

Week 47

Training tip
Many fall by the wayside, but you have persevered. Thank God for this. Strive during these last few weeks to give of your best as you race towards the finish.

Words of encouragement
Now go, and I will help you speak and will teach you what to say. Exodus 4:12

Perseverance points. Tick one block every day you do the exercises

1-10%	2-20%	3-40%	4-60%	5-80%	6-100%

THE REWARDS OF THE SPIRITUAL LIFE
The rewards will certainly not be financial—you may be less well-off as you hand over your resources to God. Yours is unlikely to be a 'life of ease' since God often demands more from his loyal servants than from others and you will lack the freedom to do as you please. Serving God does not allow that.

So what is the reward? Why make sacrifices? Why cling to God's rules?

It often seems that, in the short term, if you are corrupt, cheat, lie, "look after number one" as they say, you will do very well. Maybe. Does this mean that if you are completely honest, loving, generous and loyal, you will lose out? Materially perhaps, but that is temporary and very fickle.

God's values are not our values. There is no enduring happiness and fulfilment for the wicked. Will their apparent prosperity continue forever? Not so, says the Psalmist. Read Ps 37:8-13 and 35,36. Not so, says Jesus. Read Matt. 5:3-10, 6:19-21, 33,34, Mark 10:42-44, Luke 6:24-26.

Jesus tells us to store up our treasure in heaven. Nothing could be clearer. Would you have it any other way? Would you really want to gain the whole world and lose your soul? Forsake Jesus?

The Christian belief is that those who only 'serve' themselves in this world will in the long-term have a 'hell' of a time! This is not a cause for gloating, but great sorrow. Pray for them. Give thanks that you have been called to serve God in the way you have.

Thought for the week
The only way to get our values right is to see, not the beginning, but the end of the way, to see things not in the light of time, but in the light of eternity. William Barclay

You are the true peace of the heart, its only rest. Thomas a Kempis

WEEK 48 (& 35)

Did I . . .		Ψ	☺	TOTAL
Mon Date: Month:	253. Ψ . . . act with restraint and self-control with Jesus as my exemplary model? 254. ☺ . . . act as a counsellor? ? Listen carefully, always willing to share? [M] How can I do more to help my neighbour?	Discipline and discipleship	Right action	
Tues Date: Month:	255. Ψ . . . turn to the Lord for help when facing difficulties? 256. ☺ . . . help someone feel more at peace, feel good about themselves? [M] Who gives me the greatest moments of happiness in my life?	Faith and Friendship	Right attitude	
Wed Date: Month:	257. Ψ . . . accept sufferings as an opportunity for spiritual growth? 258. ☺ . . . give willingly when asked? Thank anyone who helped me? [M] When am I most often at fault?	Repentance and renewal	Right action	
Thur Date: Month:	259. Ψ . . . rely on God's liberality and generosity? 260. ☺ . . . avoid turning a blind eye in cases of moral wrong? [M] Where do I notice God at work?	Thanks and Trust	Right avoidance	
Fri Date: Month:	261. Ψ . . . pray the 'Lord's prayer' slowly and carefully? 262. ☺ . . . treat all with compassion, discretion, patience, and sincerity? [M] Why do I sometimes fail to hallow God's name?	Prayer and Praise	Right attitude	
Sat Date: Month:	263. Ψ . . . spend some time in contemplation? 264. ☺ . . . avoid sexual temptations, other thoughts or acts unworthy of God? [M] What thoughts do I need to control?	Learning and listening	Right avoidance	
	TOTAL WEEKLY SCORE			

Sunday weekly journal:

_____

_____

_____

_____

Week 48

Training tip

Champion athletes train their muscles hard by running up sand dunes. It's when the going gets tough and we compel ourselves to carry on that we strengthen our wills and make spiritual progress.

Words of encouragement

I wait for the LORD, my soul waits, and in his word I put my hope. Psalm 130:5

Perseverance points. Tick one block every day you do the exercises

1-10%	2-20%	3-40%	4-60%	5-80%	6-100%

GOD LOVES YOU PASSIONATELY

When we think about the love of God, it is easy to think of a cool, antiseptic kind of love that is strongly about what is best for you with some kindness thrown in. We may even imagine him sitting regally on a throne, smiling graciously at one and all but in a somewhat distant way.

Actually, we find in the Bible that God's love for his people is far from that. The images used to illustrate this love are sometimes those of a parent with a child (and those of us with children know how all-encompassing and extreme that is), and sometimes that of a man with a woman. The picture of a bridegroom and bride is often used.

I didn't know how to love God when I couldn't see him and just had to use my imagination. I felt a bit silly. So I asked God to do in me what I could not do for myself. "Please will you make me love you," I prayed. He did. When I think of him, I often get that lurch in my tummy and I tend to smile a lot. He has made me fall in love with him!

That is passionate love indeed, shot through with a lot of desire, along with enjoyment, laughter, happiness, and an urgent need to spend time together as intimately as possible.

The bible tells us that God loves us as a bridegroom loves his bride. Our love for him needs to be just as enthusiastic and overwhelming.

Thought for the week

Love is, above all, the gift of oneself. Jean Anouilh

The love of God which passeth all understanding keep your hearts and minds in the knowledge and love of God. Prayer book.

WEEK 49 (& 36)

Did I . . .		Ψ	☺	TOTAL
Mon Date: Month:	265. Ψ . . . remain still and silent before God before starting to pray? 266. ☺ . . . refuse to justify an action I should not have done? [M] Why do I do it?	Prayer and Praise	Right avoidance	
Tues Date: Month:	267. Ψ . . . study systematically rather than at random? 268. ☺ . . . use my gifts for the good of others? Do what I ought to do? [M] How can I become more serene and tranquil?	Learning and listening	Right attitude	
Wed Date: Month:	269. Ψ . . . have faith that despite my sins I was not condemned? 270. ☺ . . . put my religious or beliefs into practice? [M Where does my real passion lie?	Faith and Friendship	Right attitude	
Thur Date: Month:	271. Ψ . . . . thank God for any good I may have done? 272. ☺ . . . do a good deed? Go the extra mile to help someone? [M] When does God seem most real in my life?	Thanks and Trust	Right action	
Fri Date: Month:	273. Ψ . . . scrupulously avoid what is forbidden or dangerous? 274. ☺ . . . give a gift or compliment to someone? Point out strengths? [M] Who has influenced me most in my spiritual life?	Repentance and renewal	Right action	
Sat Date: Month:	275. Ψ . . . sacrifice my desires by putting God's will first? 276. ☺ . . . avoid miserliness, unwholesome curiosity? Refrain from resenting or envying others? [M] What mistakes do I find myself repeating?	Discipline and discipleship	Right avoidance	
	TOTAL WEEKLY SCORE			

Sunday weekly journal:

_____

_____

_____

_____

Week 49

Training tip
Keep your eyes fixed purposely on the goal. The goal is 'Victory'. 'Victory over your lower nature. Victory in fulfilling God's purpose for you in the world.

Words of encouragement
But be sure to fear the Lord, and serve him faithfully with all your heart; consider what great things he has done for you. 1 Samuel 12:24

Perseverance points. Tick one block every day you do the exercises

1-10%	2-20%	3-40%	4-60%	5-80%	6-100%

GOD IS OUR LOVER

Remember how, in the King James version of the bible, "Adam 'knew' his wife and she conceived"? Abram (Abraham) also 'knew' his wife and she conceived. The original Hebrew word for 'intercourse' and 'know' is the same (*ya'adah)*. It is a word which denotes the most intimate, tender, and loving bond possible between two people. We express something of this total self-giving when, in the Holy Eucharist, we pray "that we may evermore dwell in Him, and He in us".

Read Psalm 139. Verse 1 starts: "O LORD, you have searched me and you know me . . ." This speaks of intimacy as well as deep knowledge. There is no hiding away from God. Does this make you anxious and afraid? It shouldn't. All of us need to be found (Jesus is the Shepherd who looks for the lost sheep) and even 'found out'. God sees beyond our mistakes and failures. You are so precious to him. Psalm 139 is the joyful psalm of a person who realises what it means to be loved utterly.

Knowing you are loved is life-transforming. It energizes. It makes us more loving in return. Think what we are prepared to do to please our darling. Love is the greatest motivator we will ever know. Is there anything that is too much for God to ask of us? Is there anything that is too much for us to ask of God?

God is passionate about you—yes, you! You can trust him with all your decisions. "Cast you care on him for he cares for you" (1 Peter 5:7)

Thought for the week
Love is an act of endless forgiveness, a tender look which becomes a habit. Peter Ustinov

Holy Father, make me holy,
Holy Jesus, make me holy,
Holy Spirit, make me holy
Holy God, make me whole.—Francis Cull

WEEK 50 (& 37)

Did I . . .		Ψ	☺	**TOTAL**
Mon Date: Month:	277. Ψ . . . trust God's word in the Bible? 278. ☺ . . . persevere in doing good to all? Turn the other cheek? [M] Who needs more of my love and affection and caring?	Thanks and Trust	Right attitude	
Tues Date: Month:	279. Ψ . . . strive to know and do God's will? 280. ☺ . . . help someone? Comfort? Nurture? Assist? Make a sacrifice? [M] Why do I not trust more in God and his loving kindness and strength?	Repentance and renewal	Right action	
Wed Date: Month:	281. Ψ . . . take great comfort from the love of God? 282. ☺ . . . make people sincerely feel I had their interests at heart? [M] How can I live more simply?	Faith and Friendship	Right attitude	
Thur Date: Month:	283. Ψ . . . pray with positive expectations of guidance from the Holy Spirit? 284. ☺ . . . relentlessly fight my bad tendencies? Avoid all evil thoughts? [M] What do I do when I get stressed?	Prayer and Praise	Right avoidance	
Fri Date: Month:	285. Ψ . . . behave as I believe God wanted me to? 286. ☺ . . . avoid taking pleasure in others misfortunes? [M] When do I feel being a Christian is most worthwhile?	Discipline and discipleship	Right avoidance	
Sat Date: Month:	287. Ψ . . . increase my knowledge of God in any way? 288. ☺ . . . surprise someone with a gift of kindness? [M] Where do I want to spend the rest of my life?	Learning and listening	Right action	
	TOTAL WEEKLY SCORE			

Sunday weekly journal:

_____

_____

_____

_____

Week 50

Training tip
In any sport, from time to time you will suffer injury. In the spiritual realm, you suffer injury when you hurt others in some way. Avoid hurting others, avoid hurting yourself.

Words of encouragement
You have made known to me the path of life; you will fill me with joy in your presence, with eternal pleasure at your right hand. Psalm 16:11

Perseverance points. Tick one block every day you do the exercises

1-10%	2-20%	3-40%	4-60%	5-80%	6-100%

PURITY OF THOUGHT
St Paul warns us to fill our minds with whatever things are good and noble and worthwhile. This is sound advice, for what fills our minds eventually finds expression in our words and our lives.

It is sometimes very surprising to hear the kind of language that comes from people's mouths after surgery, or when they are delirious. Is that what was secretly stored in their minds? What would come out of your mouth or mine? I wonder.

There is a case for spending less time watching TV programmes full of violence and swearing and more watching or reading things that deal with positive things and goodness. Not that we can have no entertainment, but perhaps an evaluation of what appeals to us might be useful. The bible tells us "As a man thinks in his heart, so is he".

To deal with impure thoughts, which may arise, nip them in the bud. All of us have to face the fact that impure thoughts will arise. So far, no sin occurs. It is when we linger over them, allow them to dwell in our mind—even enjoy them!—that the trouble starts.

There are numerous techniques for dealing with this problem. One person we know presses down hard with his forefinger on the quick of his thumb whenever a bad thought arises. Ouch! This can be done quite inconspicuously. Techniques like this can work. Even better is to saturate yourself with the word of God.

Thought for the week
Faust. Unless you feel, naught will you ever gain;
Unless this feeling pours forth from your soul . . .
Goethe, Faust, I, 534

The spirit that is pure, unified and stable does not lose its inward harmony, whatever it may do, for such a spirit does everything so as to honour God, and strives to be free from all self-seeking. Thomas a Kempis

WEEK 51 (& 38)

Did I . . .		Ψ	☺	TOTAL
Mon Date: Month:	289. Ψ . . . treat my body as a holy temple? Fight the good fight? 290. ☺ . . . keep my promises and fulfil all my obligations? [M] What would make for an ideal family life?	Discipline and discipleship	Right attitude	
Tues Date: Month:	291. Ψ . . . thank God for sustenance of soul and body? 292. ☺ . . . help others not to stumble? Forgo an advantage? [M] Why do I let myself slip back from my high standards?	Thanks and Trust	Right attitude	
Wed Date: Month:	293. Ψ . . . rejoice in the Lord, enjoying my prayer time with Him? 294. ☺ . . . bless any house/workplace I entered? Pray for someone? [M] Where is the greatest need that I can do something about?	Prayer and Praise	Right action	
Thur Date: Month:	295. Ψ . . . memorise/recall any Bible passages? 296. ☺ . . . give a donation? Make amends for wrongdoing? [M] How would I live the perfect Christian life?	Learning and listening	Right action	
Fri Date: Month:	297. Ψ . . . address my predominant fault by cultivating the opposite virtue? 298. ☺ . . . keep any negative, critical or sad thoughts to myself? [M] Who needs help where I can make a difference?	Repentance and renewal	Right avoidance	
Sat Date: Month:	299. Ψ . . . maintain my faith despite problems? 300. ☺ . . . repress impure thoughts? Avoid hardness of heart or resentment? [M] When am I at my best? Worst?	Faith and Friendship	Right avoidance	
	TOTAL WEEKLY SCORE			

Sunday weekly journal:

_____

_____

_____

_____

Week 51

Training tip
You've nearly reached the end of this program. If you've completed this far you should feel enormous satisfaction. God has been working in you, you have been working for God.

Words of encouragement
Turn to me and have mercy on me, as you always do to those who love your name. Direct my footsteps according to your word; let no sin rule over me. Psalm 119: 132-133

Perseverance points. Tick one block every day you do the exercises

1-10%	2-20%	3-40%	4-60%	5-80%	6-100%

CONFIDENCE IN GOD
We know that God is a God of stupendous power. In our universe, apparently, there are a million stars for every grain of sand on earth. He is also a God of stupendous love—and he cares about each one of us.

There is a great hymn of Charles Wesley that has the verse

> Ye fearful saints, fresh courage take:
> The clouds ye so much dread
> Are thick with mercy, and will break
> In blessings on your head.

How often we forget this! How often we 'expect the worst'—as though God were not in control!

During the worst of the race riots in Johannesburg in the late 1970s, I, as a young woman, had to drop my car at the garage for a service. As I walked down the road to my office there was absolutely no one around—no cars, no pedestrians, except for a parked car with two black people in it. As I passed it, they looked at me, started the car and began to follow me. I began to quicken my pace. They came up alongside me. I was terrified. The door opened and Harriet, the cleaner at our office block, said, "Miss Margaret, would you like a lift?

Remember, no matter how alone or frightened you may feel, God is with you. Expect blessing. Expect angels to guard you. Have confidence in him. Do all he asks of you. As the concluding words of another great hymn puts it:

Love so amazing, so divine,
Demands my soul, my life my all.

Thought for the week
Be sure that if you give yourself up blindly to God's will, all will come out right, though it may seem all wrong. Do not worry, but be confident . . . Dom John Chapman

It wasn't raining when Noah built the ark. Howard Ruff

WEEK 52 (& 39)

Did I . . .		Ψ	☺	TOTAL
Mon Date: Month:	301 Ψ . . . stick to the straight and narrow? Avoid worldly ambition? 302 ☺ . . . avoid devious behaviour, covetousness? Trying to dominate? [M] When am I inclined to be judgemental or self-righteous?	Repentance and renewal	Right avoidance	
Tues Date: Month:	303 Ψ . . . give thanks for strength in time of trials? 304 ☺ . . . act with gentleness? Share privileges? [M] Where do I fall down in my spiritual life?	Thanks and Trust	Right attitude	
Wed Date: Month:	305 Ψ . . . seek guidance through books or others to help me understand God's word? 306 ☺ . . . refuse to entertain false beliefs? Avoid upsetting others? [M] Who is the best judge of my character and ability?	Learning and listening	Right avoidance	
Thur Date: Month:	307 Ψ . . . desire to make sacrifices for God? 308 ☺ . . . pray for others when I was unable to help? [M] What behaviours do I need to cultivate?	Discipline and discipleship	Right action	
Fri Date: Month:	309 Ψ . . . allow silences in my prayers waiting to hear God's voice? 310 ☺ . . . relieve others of worry, pain, distress, loss or despair? [M] How often do I read the Bible?	Prayer and Praise	Right action	
Sat Date: Month:	311 Ψ . . . hold firm to my belief that God cares about me? 312 ☺ . . . sacrifice my comfort for others? [M] Why am I certain that God is love?	Faith and Friendship	Right attitude	
	TOTAL WEEKLY SCORE			

Sunday weekly journal:

_____

_____

_____

_____

Week 52

Training tip

Congratulations. A year has gone by. You've persevered. You've learned a lot about yourself. You have formed new habits. We pray that you have grown closer to God

Words of encouragement

Blessed are they who keep his statutes and seek him with all their heart. Psalm 119:2

Perseverance points. Tick one block every day you do the exercises

1-10%	2-20%	3-40%	4-60%	5-80%	6-100%

GOOD SIGNS OF SPIRITUAL GROWTH

At the end of this year of careful thinking, praying, learning and discipline, it will help to look back to the beginning to see how you have changed and grown. God's Spirit has been at work within you, doing in you far more than you could ever imagine. Good signs are when you find yourself growing in "love, joy, peace, patience, kindness, goodness, faithfulness, gentleness and self-control."(Gal. 5.22)

Don't be upset if there are some things you expected him to deal with immediately which are still around. God has his own order of doing things and he never makes a mistake. Trust his judgment. What will have changed enormously will be your relationship with him as you have spent time with him. We rather hope you have fallen even more deeply in love with him.

Your part in your growth has been the continual opening of yourself to his grace, your determination to live only for him in every part of your life, your willingness for him to sanctify all your relationships and your acts of love and service to his people.

Now don't give up. You may want to start the year all over again. Or make a contract with yourself for more involvement. Whatever your next step will be, do find a spiritual director who will walk with you, and remember that God only works in us as we allow him to be Lord, and bring our thoughts, words and deeds under his control.

May God bless you enormously and give you his joy.

Go forward in faith:

The LORD bless you and keep you; the LORD make his face shine upon you and be gracious to you; the LORD turn his face toward you and give you peace. Numbers 6.24-26

Biblical Helps

All biblical quotes are numbered and correspond to the questions asked in terms of (1) Relationship to God and (2) Relationship to neighbor.

Week 1 and 14	Memorise?
001 Psalm 146.2: I will praise the LORD all my life; I will sing praise to my God as long as I live.	
002 Hebrews 10.24: And let us consider how we may spur one another on toward love and good deeds.	
003 Deuteronomy 6.6: These commandments that I give to you today are to be upon your hearts. Impress them on your children. Talk about them when you sit at home and when you walk along the road, when you lie down and when you get up.	
004 Colossians 3.12-14: Therefore, as God's chosen people, holy and dearly loved, clothe yourselves with compassion, kindness, humility, gentleness and patience. Bear with each other and forgive whatever grievances you may have against one another. Forgive as the Lord forgave you. And over all these virtues put on love, which binds them all together in perfect unity.	
005 Philippians 2.14-15: Do everything without complaining or arguing, so that you may become blameless and pure, children of God without fault in a crooked and depraved generation, in which you shine like stars in the universe.	
006 James 4.11-12: Brothers, do not slander one another. Anyone who speaks against his brother or judges him speaks against the law and judges it. When you judge the law, you are not keeping it, but sitting in judgment on it. There is only one Lawgiver and Judge, the one who is able to save and destroy. But you—who are you to judge your neighbor?	
007 Romans 6.23: For the wages of sin is death, but the gift of God is eternal life in Christ Jesus our Lord.	
008 Leviticus 25.43: Do not rule over them ruthlessly, but fear your God.	
009 Romans 10.17: Consequently, faith comes from hearing the message, and the message is heard through the word of Christ.	

	Memorise?
010 Numbers 6.24-26: The LORD bless you and keep you; the LORD make his face shine upon you and be gracious to you; the LORD turn his face toward you and give you peace	
011 John 15.13: Greater love has no one than this, that he lay down his life for his friends.	
012 1 Peter 3.9: Do not repay evil with evil or insult with insult, but with blessing, because to this you were called so that you may inherit a blessing.	
Week 2 and 15	**Memorise?**
013 Hebrews 11.6: And without faith it is impossible to please God, because anyone who comes to him must believe that he exists and that he rewards those who earnestly seek him.	
014 Proverbs 16.24: Pleasant words are a honeycomb, sweet to the soul and healing to the bones.	
015 1 John 1.6-7: If we claim to have fellowship with him yet walk in the darkness, we lie and do not live by the truth. But if we walk in the light, as he is the light, we have fellowship with one another, and the blood of Jesus, his Son, purifies us from all sin.	
016 1 John 4.11: Dear friends, since God so loved us, we also ought to love one another.	
017 1 Corinthians 14.12: Since you are eager to have spiritual gifts, try to excel in gifts that build up the church.	
018 Matthew 7.2: For in the same way you judge others, you will be judged, and with the measure you use, it will be measured to you.	
019 Matthew 21.22: If you believe, you will receive whatever you ask for in prayer.	
020 Romans 14.12: So then, each of us will give an account of himself to God.	
021 Jeremiah 17.7-8: "But blessed is the man who trusts in the LORD, whose confidence is in him. He will be like a tree planted by the water that sends out its roots by the stream. It does not fear when heat comes; its leaves are always green. It has no worries in a year of drought and never fails to bear fruit."	
022 Proverbs 3.27: Do not withhold good from those who deserve it, when it is in your power to act.	
023 2 Timothy 3.16-17: All Scripture is God-breathed and is useful for teaching, rebuking, correcting and training in righteousness, so that the man of God may be thoroughly equipped for every good work.	
024 Ephesians 4.29: Do not let any unwholesome talk come out of your mouths, but only what is helpful for building others up according to their needs, that it may benefit those who listen.	
Week 3 and 16	**Memorise?**
025 Luke 3.9: " . . . and every tree that does not produce good fruit will be cut down and thrown into the fire."	

026 Isaiah 42.20 You have seen many things, but have paid no attention; your ears are open, but you hear nothing.	
027 Psalm 9.1-2: I will praise you, O LORD, with all my heart; I will tell of all your wonders. I will be glad and rejoice in you; I will sing praise to your name, O Most High.	
028 James 3.18: Peacemakers who sow in peace raise a harvest of righteousness.	
029 James 1.19: Everyone should be quick to listen . . .	
030 Luke 6.41: Why do you look at the speck of sawdust in your brother's eye and pay no attention to the plank in your own eye?	
031 Colossians 3.15: Let the peace of Christ rule in your hearts, since as members of one body you were called to peace. And be thankful.	
032 Proverbs 19.11: A man's wisdom gives him patience; it is to his glory to overlook an offense.	
033 2 Timothy 3.2-5: People will be lovers of themselves, lovers of money, boastful, proud, abusive, disobedient to their parents, ungrateful, unholy without love, unforgiving, slanderous, without self-control, brutal, not lovers of the good, treacherous, rash, conceited, lovers of pleasure rather than lovers of God—having a form of godliness but denying its power. Have nothing to do with them.	
034 Nehemiah 9.17: . . . But you are a forgiving God, gracious and compassionate, slow to anger and abounding in love	
035 Isaiah 1.18: "Come now, let us reason together," says the LORD.	
036 Matthew 5.16: In the same way, let your light shine before men, that they may see your good deeds and praise your Father in heaven.	
Week 4 and 17	Memorise?
037 James 4.17: Anyone, then, who knows the good he ought to do and doesn't do it, sins.	
038 Proverbs 30.32: If you have played the fool and exalted yourself, or if you have planned evil, clap your hand over your mouth!	
039 James 1.2-4: Consider it pure joy, my brothers, whenever you face trials of many kinds, because you know that the testing of your faith develops perseverance. Perseverance must finish its work so that you may be mature and complete, not lacking anything.	
040 Matthew 19.19: . . . honor your father and mother and 'love your neighbor as yourself.'	
041 1 Corinthians 10.31: So whether you eat or drink or whatever you do, do it all for the glory of God.	
042 1 Corinthians 10.24: Nobody should seek his own good, but the good of others.	
043 1 Corinthians 14.15: So what shall I do? I will pray with my spirit, but I will also pray with my mind; I will sing with my spirit, but I will also sing with my mind.	

044 Proverbs 16.7-8: When a man's ways are pleasing to the LORD, he makes even his enemies live at peace with him. Better a little with righteousness than much gain with injustice.	
045 Psalm 81.11-12: But my people would not listen to me; Israel would not submit to me. So I gave them over to their own stubborn hearts to follow their own devices.	
046 Hebrews 13.17: Obey your leaders and submit to their authority.	
047 Acts 17.28: For in him we live and move and have our being.	
048 Romans 15.1-2: We who are strong ought to bear with the failings of the weak and not to please ourselves. Each of us should please his neighbor for his good, to build him up.	
Week 5 and 18	Memorise?
049 Proverbs 4.1-2: Listen, my sons, to a father's instruction; pay attention and gain understanding. I give you sound learning, so do not forsake my teaching.	
050 Luke 6.36-38: Be merciful, just as your Father is merciful. Do not judge, and you will not be judged. Do not condemn, and you will not be condemned. Forgive, and you will be forgiven. Give, and it will be given to you . . .	
051 1 Timothy 6.6-7: But godliness with contentment is great gain. For we brought nothing into the world, and we can take nothing out of it.	
052 Mark 7.21: For from within, out of men's hearts, come evil thoughts, sexual immorality, theft, murder, adultery, greed, malice, deceit, lewdness, envy, slander, arrogance and folly.	
053 James 5.16: Therefore confess your sins to each other and pray for each other so that you may be healed. The prayer of a righteous man is powerful and effective.	
054 Psalm 106.3: Blessed are they who maintain justice, who constantly do what is right.	
055 Romans 1.16: I am not ashamed of the gospel, because it is the power of God for the salvation of everyone who believes; first for the Jew, then for the Gentile.	
056 1 Peter 1.22: Now that you have purified yourselves by obeying the truth so that you have sincere love for your brothers, love one another deeply, from the heart.	
057 Ephesians 3.20-21: Now to him who is able to do immeasurably more than all we can ask or imagine, according to his power that is at work within us, to him be glory in the church and in Christ Jesus throughout all generations, for ever and ever! Amen.	
058 Romans 14.19: Let us therefore make every effort to do what leads to peace and to mutual edification.	
059 James 1.13-14: . . . For God cannot be tempted by evil, nor does he tempt anyone; but each one is tempted when, by his own evil desire, he is dragged away and enticed.	

060 1 John 3.17: If anyone has material possessions and sees his brother in need but has no pity on him, how can the love of God be in him?	
Week 6 and 19	Memorise?
061 Isaiah 26.4: Trust in the LORD forever, for the LORD, the LORD, is the Rock eternal.	
062 Psalm 12.2: Everyone lies to his neighbor; their flattering lips speak with deception.	
063 John 7: 16-17: Jesus answered, "My teaching is not my own. It comes from him who sent me. If anyone chooses to do God's will, he will find out whether my teaching comes from God or whether I speak on my own."	
064 1 Peter 2.1: Therefore, rid yourself of all malice and all deceit, hypocrisy, envy and slander of every kind.	
065 Matthew 17.20: " . . . I tell you the truth, if you have faith as small as a mustard seed you can say to this mountain, 'Move from here to there' and it will move. Nothing will be impossible for you."	
066 Acts 20.35: In everything I did, I showed you that by this kind of hard work we must help the weak, remembering the words of the Lord Jesus himself said: 'It is more blessed to give than to receive.'	
067 1 Corinthians 4.2: Now it is required that those who have been given a trust must prove faithful.	
068 Proverbs 4.13-14: Hold on to instruction, do not let it go; guard it well, for it is your life. Do not set foot on the path of the wicked or walk in the way of evil men.	
069 2 Kings 20.5: . . . I have heard your prayer and seen your tears; I will heal you.	
070 1 John 4.7-8: Dear friends, let us love one another, for love comes from God. Everyone who loves has been born of God and knows God. Whoever does not love does not know God, because God is love.	
071 Matthew 5.44-45: But I tell you: Love your enemies and pray for those who persecute you, that you may be sons of your Father who is in heaven . . .	
072 Proverbs 14.21: He who despises his neighbor sins, but blessed is he who is kind to the needy.	
Week 7 and 20	Memorise?
073 Luke 6.12: One of those days Jesus went out to a mountainside to pray, and spent the night praying to God.	
074 James 4.8: Come near to God and he will come near to you. Wash your hands, you sinners, and purify your hearts, you double-minded.	
075 Luke 13.24: "Make every effort to enter through the narrow door, because many, I tell you, will try to enter and will not be able to."	
076 Matthew 5.41: If someone forces you to go one mile, go with him two miles.	

077 Proverbs 30.5-6: Every word of God is flawless; he is a shield to those who take refuge in him. Do not add to his words, or he will rebuke you and prove you a liar.	
078 Luke 6.31: Do to others as you would have them do to you.	
079 Psalm 35.18: I will give you thanks in the great assembly; among throngs of people I will praise you.	
080 Matthew 5.22: But I tell you that anyone who is angry with his brother will be subject to judgment . . .	
081 1 John 1.9-10: If we confess our sins, he is faithful and just and will forgive us our sins and purify us from all unrighteousness. If we claim we have not sinned, we make him out to be a liar and his word has no place in our lives.	
082 Proverbs 12.25: An anxious heart weighs a man down, but a kind word cheers him up.	
083 Philippians 1.27: Whatever happens, conduct yourselves in a manner worthy of the gospel of Christ . . .	
084 Matthew 5.42: Give to the one who asks you, and do not turn away from the one who wants to borrow from you.	
Week 8 and 21	Memorise?
085 Psalm 37.40. The LORD helps them and delivers them; he delivers them from the wicked and saves them, because they take refuge in him.	
086 Romans 14.13: Therefore let us stop passing judgment on one another. Instead, make up your mind not to put any stumbling block or obstacle in your brother's way.	
087 Joel 2.13: Rend your heart and not your garments. Return to the LORD your God, for he is gracious and compassionate, slow to anger and abounding in love . . .	
088 1 John 3.18: Dear children, let us not love with words or tongue but with actions and in truth.	
089 Matthew 12.25: Jesus knew their thoughts and said to them, "Every kingdom divided against itself will be ruined, and every city or household divided against itself will not stand."	
090 Hosea 10.12: Sow for yourselves righteousness, reap the fruit of unfailing love, and break up your unplowed ground; for it is time to seek the LORD, until he comes and showers righteousness on you.	
091 1 Peter 1.14-16: As obedient children, do not conform to the evil desires you had when you lived in ignorance. But just as he who called you is holy, so be holy in all you do; for it is written: "Be holy, because I am holy."	
092 Matthew 5.14: You are the light of the world.	
093 James 4.2-3: . . . You do not have, because you do not ask God. When you ask, you do not receive, because you ask with wrong motives, that you may spend what you get on your pleasures.	

	Memorise?
094 Colossians 4.5-6: Be wise in the way you act toward outsiders; make the most of every opportunity. Let your conversation be always full of grace, seasoned with salt, so that you may know how to answer everyone.	
095 Deuteronomy 6.5: Love the LORD your God with all your heart and with all your soul and with all your strength.	
096 2 Corinthians 4.2: Rather, we have renounced secret and shameful ways; we do not use deception, nor do we distort the word of God. On the contrary, by setting forth the truth plainly we commend ourselves to every man's conscience in the sight of God.	
Week 9 and 22	Memorise?
097 Luke 9.47-48: Jesus, knowing their thoughts, took a little child and had him stand beside him. Then he said to them, "Whoever welcomes this little child in my name welcomes me; and whoever welcomes me welcomes the one who sent me." . . .	
098 Job 6.14: A despairing man should have the devotion of his friends, even though he forsakes the fear of the Almighty.	
099 Matthew 6.7-8: And when you pray, do not keep on babbling like pagans, for they think they will be heard because of their many words. Do not be like them, for your Father knows what you need before you ask him.	
100 Romans 12.21: Do not be overcome by evil, but overcome evil with good.	
101 Revelations 7.11-12: . . . They fell down on their faces before the throne and worshipped God, saying; "Amen! Praise and glory and wisdom and thanks and honor and power and strength be to our God for ever and ever. Amen!"	
102 Titus 3.1-2: Remind the people to be subject to rulers and authorities, to be obedient, to be ready to do whatever is good, to slander no one, to be peaceable and considerate, and to show true humility toward all men.	
103 Lamentations 3.25-26: The LORD is good to those whose hope is in him, to the one who seeks him; it is good to wait quietly for the salvation of the LORD.	
104 Matthew 15.11: What goes into a man's mouth does not make him 'unclean,' but what comes out of his mouth, that is what makes him 'unclean.'	
105 Matthew 11.29: "Take my yoke upon you and learn from me, for I am gentle and humble in heart, and you will find rest for your souls. For my yoke is easy and my burden is light."	
106 Proverbs 31.8: Speak up for those who cannot speak for themselves . . .	
107 Hebrews 3.12: See to it, brothers, that none of you has a sinful, unbelieving heart that turns away from the living God.	
108 Proverbs 21.21: He who pursues righteousness and love finds life, prosperity and honor.	

Week 10 and 23	Memorise?
109 Philippians 4.8: Finally, brothers, whatever is true, whatever is noble, whatever is right, whatever is pure, whatever is lovely, whatever is admirable—if anything is excellent or praiseworthy—think about such things.	
110 Luke 17.10: So you also, when you have done everything you were told to do, should say, 'We are unworthy servants; we have only done our duty.'	
111 Psalm 32.8: I will instruct you and teach you in the way you should go; I will counsel you and watch over you.	
112 Proverbs 6.16-19: There are six things the LORD hates, seven that are detestable to him: haughty eyes, a lying tongue, hands that shed innocent blood, a heart that devises wicked schemes, feet that are quick to rush into evil, a false witness who pours out lies, and a man who stirs up dissension among brothers.	
113 Ephesians 5.19-20: Speak to one another with psalms, hymns and spiritual songs. Sing and make music in your heart to the Lord, always giving thanks to God the Father for everything, in the name of our Lord Jesus Christ.	
114 Proverbs 11.1: The LORD abhors dishonest scales, but accurate weights are his delight.	
115 Hebrews 2.1: We must pay more careful attention, therefore, to what we have heard, so that we do not drift away.	
116 Psalm 119.37: Turn my eyes from worthless things; preserve my life according to your word.	
117 1 Peter 3.17: It is better, if it is God's will, to suffer for doing good than for doing evil.	
118 Hebrews 12.14: Make every effort to live in peace with all men and to be holy; without holiness no one will see the Lord.	
119 Ecclesiastes 5.1-2: Guard your steps when you go to the house of God. Go near to listen rather than to offer the sacrifice of fools, who do not know that they do wrong. Do not be quick with your mouth, do not be hasty in your heart to utter anything before God. God is in heaven and you are on earth, so let your words be few.	
120 Daniel 4.27: . . . Renounce your sins by doing what is right, and your wickedness by being kind to the oppressed. It may be that then your prosperity will continue.	
Week 11 and 24	Memorise?
121 Psalm 19.1: The heavens declare the glory of God; the skies proclaim the work of his hands.	
122 Colossians 3.23: Whatever you do, work at it with all your heart, as working for the Lord, not for men . . .	
123 Psalm 103.1: Praise the LORD, O my soul; all my inmost being, praise his holy name.	

	Memorise?
124 Matthew 25.35: For I was hungry and you gave me something to eat, I was thirsty and you gave me something to drink, I was a stranger and you invited me in	
125 Mark 16.15: He said to them, "Go into all the world and preach the good news to all creation."	
126 Hosea 12.6: But you must return to your God, maintain love and justice, and wait for your God always.	
127 Psalm 131.1-2: My heart is not proud, O LORD, my eyes are not haughty; I do not concern myself with great matters or things too wonderful for me. But I have stilled and quieted my soul; like a weaned child with its mother, like a weaned child is my soul within me.	
128 1 Timothy 5.8: If anyone does not provide for his relatives, and especially for his immediate family, he has denied the faith and is worse than an unbeliever.	
129 Psalm 18.30 As for God, his way is perfect; the word of the LORD is flawless. He is a shield for all who take refuge in him.	
130 Ephesians 4.31-32: Get rid of all bitterness, rage and anger, brawling and slander, along with every form of malice. Be kind and compassionate to one another, forgiving each other, just as in Christ God forgave you.	
131 James 4.7: Submit yourselves, then, to God. Resist the devil, and he will flee from you.	
132 Ephesians 5.15-17: Be very careful, then, how you live—not as unwise but as wise, making the most of every opportunity, because the days are evil. Therefore do not be foolish, but understand what the Lord's will is.	
Week 12 and 25	Memorise?
133 2 Timothy 4.3-4: For the time will come when men will not put up with sound doctrine. Instead, to suit their own desires, they will gather around them a great number of teachers to say what their itching ears want to hear. They will turn their ears away from the truth and turn aside to myths.	
134 Proverbs 12.20: There is deceit in the hearts of those who plot evil, but joy for those who promote peace.	
135 Luke 11.17: Jesus knew their thoughts and said to them: "Any kingdom divided against itself will be ruined, and a house divided against itself will fall."	
136 James 5.9: Don't grumble against each other, brothers, or you will be judged. The Judge is standing at the door!	
137 2 Peter 3.14: So then, dear friends, since you are looking forward to this, make every effort to be found spotless, blameless and at peace with him.	
138 John 14.27: Peace I leave with you; my peace I give you . . .	
139 Romans 8.35: Who shall separate us from the love of Christ? Shall trouble or hardship or persecution or famine or nakedness or danger or sword?	

140 Ecclesiastes 12.14: For God will bring every deed into judgment, including every hidden thing, whether it is good or evil.	
141 Colossians 1.9 For this reason, since the day we heard about you, we have not stopped praying for you and asking God to fill you with the knowledge of his will through all spiritual wisdom and understanding.	
142 Job 4.6: Should not your piety be your confidence and your blameless ways your hope?	
143 Matthew 6.19-21. "Do not store up for yourselves treasures on earth, where moth and rust destroy, and where thieves break in and steal. But store up for yourselves treasures in heaven . . . For where your treasure is, there your heart will be also.	
144 Hebrews 13.16: And do not forget to do good and to share with others, for with such sacrifices God is pleased.	
Week 13 and 26	Memorise?
145 Hebrews 13.15: Through Jesus, therefore, let us continually offer to God a sacrifice of praise—the fruit of lips that confess his name.	
146 John 13.34: A new command I give you: Love one another. As I have loved you, so you must love one another.	
147 Psalm 32.5: Then I acknowledged my sin to you and did not cover up my iniquity. I said, "I will confess my transgressions to the LORD"—and you forgave the guilt of my sin.	
148 Jeremiah 39.12: Take him and look after him; don't harm him but do for him whatever he asks.	
149 Psalm 19.8: The precepts of the LORD are right, giving joy to the heart. The commands of the LORD are radiant, giving light to the eyes.	
150 Romans 12.17-18: Do not repay anyone evil for evil. Be careful to do what is right in the eyes of everybody. If it is possible, as far as it depends on you, live at peace with everyone.	
151 Galatians 4.6: Because you are sons, God sent the Spirit of his Son into our hearts, the Spirit who calls out, "*Abba*, Father." So you are no longer a slave, but a son; and since you are a son, God has made you also an heir.	
152 James 1.26-27: If anyone considers himself religious and yet does not keep a tight rein on his tongue, he deceives himself and his religion is worthless. Religion that God our Father accepts as pure and faultless is this: to look after orphans and widows in their distress and to keep oneself from being polluted by the world.	
153 Psalm 119.133: Direct my footsteps according to your word, let no sin rule over me.	
154 Proverbs 20.3: It is to a man's honor to avoid strife, but every fool is quick to quarrel.	
155 1 Thessalonians 5.16-18: Be joyful always; pray continually; give thanks in all circumstances, for this is God's will for you in Christ Jesus.	

156 2 Timothy 2.24: And the Lord's servant must not quarrel; instead, he must be kind to everyone, able to teach, not resentful.	
Week 27 and 40	Memorise?
157 Psalm 127.1: Unless the LORD builds the house, its builders labor in vain.	
158 Proverbs 17.22: A cheerful heart is good medicine, but a crushed spirit dries up the bones.	
159 Psalm 47.7: For God is the King of all the earth; sing to him a psalm of praise.	
160 1 Timothy 6.10: For the love of money is a root of all kinds of evil. Some people, eager for money, have wandered from the faith and pierced themselves with many griefs.	
161 Luke 14.27: And anyone who does not carry his cross and follow me cannot be my disciple.	
162 1 Corinthians 13.11: When I was a child, I talked like a child, I thought like a child, I reasoned like a child. When I became a man, I put childish ways behind me.	
163 Psalm 119.24: Your statutes are my delight; they are my counsellors.	
164 Matthew 6.34 :Therefore do not worry about tomorrow, for tomorrow will worry about itself. Each day has enough trouble of its own.	
165 Matthew 7.7: "Ask and it will be given to you; seek and you will find; knock and the door will be opened to you. For everyone who asks receives; he who seeks finds; and to him who knocks, the door will be opened."	
166 Romans 2.6: God "will give to each person according to what he has done."	
167 Luke 16.10: Whoever can be trusted with very little can also be trusted with much, and whoever is dishonest with very little will also be dishonest with much.	
168 1 Peter 2.12: Live such good lives among the pagans that, though they accuse you of doing wrong, they may see your good deeds and glorify God on the day he visits us.	
Week 28 and 41	Memorise?
169 Psalm 1.1-2: Blessed is the man who does not walk in the counsel of the wicked or stand in the way of sinners or sit in the seat of mockers.	
170 Proverbs 25.6-7: Do not exalt yourself in the king's presence, and do not claim a place among great men; it is better for him to say to you, "Come up here," than for him to humiliate you before a nobleman.	
171 Matthew 5.8: Blessed are the pure in heart, for they will see God.	
172 James 1.17-18: Every good and perfect gift is from above, coming down from the Father of the heavenly lights, who does not change like shifting shadows.	

	Memorise?
173 Isaiah 41.10: So do not fear, for I am with you; do not be dismayed, for I am your God. I will strengthen you and help you; I will uphold you with my righteous hand.	
174 Luke 10.35: The next day he took out two silver coins and gave them to the innkeeper. 'Look after him,' he said, 'and when I return, I will reimburse you for any extra expense you may have.'	
175 : Then Jesus told his disciples a parable to show them that they should always pray and not give up.	
176 Titus 1.7-8: Since an overseer is entrusted with God's work, he must be blameless—not over-bearing, not quick-tempered, not given to drunkenness, not violent, not pursuing dishonest gain. Rather he must be hospitable, one who loves what is good, who is self-controlled, upright, holy and disciplined.	
177 Proverbs 4.4: . . . he taught me and said, "Lay hold of my words with all your heart; keep my commands and you will live."	
178 Proverbs 11.24: One man gives freely, yet gains even more; another withholds unduly, but comes to poverty	
179 Daniel 6.10: Now when Daniel heard that the decree had been published, he went home to his upstairs room where the windows opened toward Jerusalem. Three times a day he got down on his knees and prayed, giving thanks to his God	
180 Job 5.8: But if it were I, I would appeal to God; I would lay my cause before him.	
Week 29 and 42	Memorise?
181 Romans 8.26: In the same way, the Spirit helps us in our weakness. We do not know what we ought to pray for, but the Spirit himself intercedes for us with groans that words cannot express.	
182 Proverbs 12.18: Reckless words pierce like a sword, but the tongue of the wise brings healing.	
183 Psalm 119.78: May the arrogant be put to shame for wronging me without cause; but I will meditate on your precepts.	
184 Ephesians 4.22-24: You were taught, with regard to your former way of life, to put off your old self, which is being corrupted by its deceitful desires; to be made new in the attitude of your minds; and to put on the new self, created to be like God in true righteousness and holiness.	
185 Matthew 7.11 If you, then, though you are evil, know how to give good gifts to your children, how much more will your Father in heaven give good gifts to those who ask him!	
186 Matthew 6.3-4: But when you give to the needy, do not let your left hand know what your right hand is doing, so that your giving may be in secret. Then your Father, who sees what is done in secret, will reward you.	
187 James 1.6-7: But when he asks, he must believe and not doubt, because he who doubts is like a wave of the sea, blown and tossed by the wind. That man should not think he will receive anything from the Lord; he is a double-minded man, unstable in all he does.	

	Memorise?
188 Proverbs 24.29: Do not say, "I'll do to him as he has done to me; I'll pay that man back for what he did."	
189 James 2.23: And the scripture was fulfilled that says, "Abraham believed God, and it was credited to him as righteousness," and he was called God's friend.	
190 Romans 14.7-8: For none of us lives to himself alone and none of us dies to himself alone. If we live, we live to the Lord; and if we die, we die to the Lord.	
191 Romans 8.28: And we know that in all things God works for the good of those who love him, who have been called according to his purpose.	
192 2 Timothy 2.15-16: Do your best to present yourself to God as one approved, a workman who does not need to be ashamed and who correctly handles the word of truth. Avoid godless chatter, because those who indulge in it will become more and more ungodly.	
Week 30 and 43	Memorise?
193 Proverbs 28.20: A faithful man will be richly blessed, but one eager to get rich will not go unpunished.	
194 Matthew 6.14-15: For if you forgive men when they sin against you, your heavenly Father will also forgive you. But if you do not forgive men their sins, your Father will not forgive your sins.	
195 John 6.27: Do not work for food that spoils, but for food that endures to eternal life, which the Son of Man will give you. On him God the Father has placed his seal of approval.	
196 Proverbs 25.28: Like a city whose walls are broken down is a man who lacks self-control.	
197 Hebrews 13.5: Keep your lives free from the love of money and be content with what you have . . .	
198 1 Samuel 2.3: "Do not keep talking so proudly or let your mouth speak such arrogance, for the LORD is a God who knows, and by him deeds are weighed.	
199 Proverbs 20.27: The lamp of the LORD searches the spirit of a man; it searches out his inmost being.	
200 Matthew 12.34-35: . . . For out of the overflow of the heart the mouth speaks. The good man brings good things out of the good stored up in him, and the evil man brings evil things out of the evil stored up in him.	
201 Psalm 106.1-2: . . . Give thanks to the LORD, for he is good; his love endures forever. Who can proclaim the mighty acts of the LORD or fully declare his praise?	
202 Ephesians 4.25-27: Therefore each of you must put off falsehood and speak truthfully to his neighbor, for we are all members of one body. In your anger do not sin; do not let the sun go down while you are still angry, and do not give the devil a foothold.	

	Memorise?
203 Matthew 6.1 Be careful not to do your 'acts of righteousness' before men, to be seen by them. If you do, you will have no reward from your Father in heaven.	
204 2 Corinthians 9.10-11: Now he who supplies seed to the sower and bread for food will also supply and increase your store of seed and will enlarge the harvest of your righteousness. You will be made rich in every way so that you can be generous on every occasion, and through us your generosity will result in thanksgiving to God.	
Week 31 and 44	**Memorise?**
205 Matthew 6.31-33: So do not worry, saying, 'What shall we eat?' or 'What shall we drink?' or 'What shall we wear?' For the pagans run after all these things, and your heavenly Father knows that you need them. But seek first his kingdom and his righteousness, and all these things will be given to you as well.	
206 Jeremiah 7.23: . . . but I gave them this command: Obey me and I will be your God and you will be my people. Walk in all the ways that I command you, that it may go well with you	
207 1 John 2.3-4: We know that we have come to know him if we obey his commands. The man who says, "I know him," but does not do what he commands is a liar, and the truth is not in him.	
208 Matthew 7.12: So in everything, do to others what you would have them do to you, for this sums up the Law and the Prophets.	
209 Isaiah 30.21: Whether you turn to the right or to the left, your ears will hear a voice behind you, saying, "this is the way; walk in it."	
210 2 Corinthians 6.4 . . . 7: Rather, as servants of God we commend ourselves in every way: in great endurance; in troubles, hardships and distresses . . . in the Holy Spirit and in sincere love; in truthful speech and in the power of God . . .	
211 Psalm 23. 1-3: The LORD is my shepherd, I shall not be in want. He makes me lie down in green pastures, he leads me beside quiet waters, he restores my soul.	
212 Hebrews 13.1-2: Keep on loving each other as brothers. Do not forget to entertain strangers, for by so doing some people have entertained angels without knowing it.	
213 Matthew 5.48: Be perfect, therefore, as your heavenly Father is perfect.	
214 Proverbs 6.6: Go the ant, you sluggard; consider its ways and be wise.	
215 John 14.6: Jesus answered, "I am the way and the truth and the life. No one comes to the Father except through me.	
216 Proverbs 11.12: A man who lacks judgment derides his neighbor, but a man of understanding holds his tongue.	
Week 32 and 45	**Memorise?**
217 Matthew 18.6: But if anyone causes one of these little ones who believe in me to sin, it would be better for him to have a large millstone hung around his neck and to be drowned in the depths of the sea.	

	Memorise?
218 Job 34.4: Let us discern for ourselves what is right; let us learn together what is good.	
219 2 Corinthians 4.8-10: We are hard pressed on every side, but not crushed; perplexed, but not in despair; persecuted, but not abandoned; struck down, but not destroyed. We always carry around in our body the death of Jesus, so that the life of Jesus may also be revealed in our body.	
220 Job 5.17: Blessed is the man whom God corrects; so do not despise the discipline of the Almighty.	
221 Philippians 2.10-11: . . . that at the name of Jesus every knee should bow, in heaven and on earth and under the earth, and every tongue confess that Jesus Christ is Lord, to the glory of God the Father.	
222 Matthew 25.40: The King will reply, 'I tell you the truth, whatever you did for one of the least of these my brothers of mine, you did to me.'	
223 2 Timothy 1.7: For God did not give us a spirit of timidity, but a spirit of power, of love and of self-discipline.	
224 Matthew 22.21: . . . Then he said to them, "Give to Caesar what is Caesar's, and to God what is God's."	
225 Proverbs 12.15: The way of a fool seems right to him, but a wise man listens to advice.	
226 Matthew 23.12: For whoever exalts himself will be humbled, and whoever humbles himself will be exalted.	
227 Psalm 63.8: My soul clings to you; your right hand upholds me.	
228 Luke 6.27-28: But I tell you who hear me: Love your enemies, do good to those who hate you, bless those who curse you, pray for those who mistreat you.	
Week 33 and 46	Memorise?
229 Numbers 12.6: . . . he said, "Listen to my words: "When a prophet of the LORD is among you, I reveal myself to him in visions, I speak to him in dreams . . ."	
230 Hebrews 13.4: Marriage should be honored by all, and the marriage bed kept pure, for God will judge the adulterer, and all the sexually immoral.	
231 Joshua 24.14: Now fear the LORD and serve him with all faithfulness.	
232 Proverbs 15.28: The heart of the righteous weighs its answers, but the mouth of the wicked gushes evil.	
233 Romans 12.1: Therefore, I urge you, brothers, in view of God's mercy, to offer your bodies as living sacrifices, holy and pleasing to God—this is your spiritual act of worship.	
234 Romans 12.9-11: Love must be sincere. Hate what is evil; cling to what is good. Be devoted to one another in brotherly love. Never be lacking in zeal, but keep your spiritual fervor, serving the Lord.	
235 Proverbs 3.5: Trust in the LORD with all your heart and lean not on your own understanding.	

236 Mark 3.35: Whoever does God's will is my brother and sister and mother.	
237 Mark 10.21 Jesus looked at him and loved him	
238 1 Thessalonians 4.7-8: For God did not call us to be impure, but to live a holy life. Therefore, he who rejects this instruction does not reject man but God, who gives you his Holy Spirit.	
239 James 3.16-17 : For where you have envy and selfish ambition, there you find disorder and every evil practice. But the wisdom that comes from heaven is first of all pure; then peace-loving, considerate, submissive, full of mercy and good fruit, impartial and sincere.	
240 Psalm 139.23: Search me, O God, and know my heart; test me and know my anxious thoughts.	
Week 34 and 47	Memorise?
241 Philippians 4.13: I can do everything through him who gives me strength.	
242 Colossians 3.8: But now you must rid yourselves of all such things as these: anger, rage, malice, slander, and filthy language from your lips.	
243 Proverbs 19.21: Many are the plans in a man's heart, but it is the LORD'S purpose that prevails.	
244 1 Corinthians 13. 4-7: Love is patient, love is kind. It does not envy, it does not boast, it is not proud. It is not rude, it is not self-seeking, it is not easily angered. It keeps no record of wrongs. Love does not delight in evil but rejoices with the truth. It always protects, always trusts, always hopes, always perseveres.	
245 Proverbs 1.33: . . . but whoever listens to me will live in safety and be at ease, without fear of harm.	
246 1 Thessalonians 5.14-15: And we urge you, brothers, warn those who are idle, encourage the timid, help the weak, be patient with everyone. Make sure that nobody pays back wrong for wrong, but always try to be kind to each other and to everyone else.	
247 Jeremiah 29.11: "For I know the plans I have for you," declares the LORD, "plans to prosper you and not to harm you, plans to give you hope and a future."	
248 2 Corinthians 9.6-7: Remember this: Whoever sows sparingly will also reap sparingly, and whoever sows generously will also reap generously. Each man should give what he has decided in his heart to give, not reluctantly or under compulsion, for God loves a cheerful giver.	
249 1 Peter 5.7: Cast all your anxiety on him because he cares for you.	
250 Deuteronomy 30.19: . . . I have set before you life and death, blessings and curses. Now choose life . . .	
251 1 John 5.14-15: This is the confidence we have in approaching God: that if we ask anything according to his will, he hears us. And if we know that he hears us—whatever we ask—we know that we have what we have asked of him.	

252 Jeremiah 17.9: The heart is deceitful above all things and beyond cure. Who can understand it?	
Week 35 and 48	Memorise?
253 1 Corinthians 4.12-13: . . . When we are cursed, we bless; when we are persecuted, we endure it; when we are slandered, we answer kindly	
254 199 Isaiah 41.28: I look but there is no one—no one among them to give counsel, no one to give answer when I ask them.	
255 Matthew 11.28: Come to me, all you who are weary and burdened, and I will give you rest.	
256 Matthew 5.5: Blessed are the meek, for they will inherit the earth.	
257 Romans 8.18: I consider that our present sufferings are not worth comparing with the glory that will be revealed in us.	
258 Lamentations 4.4: Because of thirst the infant's tongue sticks to the roof of its mouth; the children beg for bread, but no one gives it to them.	
259 Hebrews 4.16: Let us then approach the throne of grace with confidence, so that we may receive mercy and find grace to help us in our time of need.	
260 Jeremiah 22.3: This is what the LORD says: Do what is just and right. Rescue from the hand of his oppressor the one who has been robbed. Do no wrong or violence to the alien, the fatherless or the widow, and do not shed innocent blood in this place.	
261 Colossians 4.2: Devote yourselves to prayer, being watchful and thankful.	
262 Proverbs 19.17: He who is kind to the poor lends to the LORD, and he will reward him for what he has done	
263 Luke 2.19: But Mary treasured up all these things and pondered them in her heart.	
264 Romans 6.12: Therefore do not let sin reign in your mortal body so that you obey its evil desires.	
Week 36 and 49	Memorise?
265 Psalm 27.4: One thing I ask of the LORD, this is what I seek; that I may dwell in the house of the LORD all the days of my life, to gaze upon the beauty of the LORD and to seek him in his temple.	
266 Romans 7.20: Now if I do what I do not want to do, it is no longer I who do it, but it is sin living in me that does it.	
267 1 Thessalonians 4.1: Finally, brothers, we instructed you how to live in order to please God, as in fact you are living. Now we ask you and urge you in the Lord Jesus to do this more and more.	
268 2 Peter 1.5-7: For this reason, make every effort to add to your faith goodness; and to goodness, knowledge; and to knowledge, self-control; and to self-control, perseverance; and to perseverance, godliness; and to godliness, brotherly kindness; and to brotherly kindness, love.	

	Memorise?
269 Romans 8.1-2: Therefore, there is now no condemnation for those who are in Christ Jesus, because through Christ Jesus the law of the Spirit of life set me free from the law of sin and death.	
270 James 2.15-16: Suppose a brother or sister is without clothes and daily food. If one of you says to him, "Go, I wish you well; keep warm and well fed," but does nothing about his physical needs, what good is it?	
271 Luke 6.35: But love your enemies, do good to them, and lend to them without expecting to get anything back. Then your reward will be great, and you will be sons of the most High, because he is kind to the ungrateful and wicked.	
272 Matthew 16.26-27: What good will it be for a man if he gains the whole world, yet forfeits his soul? Or what can a man give in exchange for his soul? For the Son of Man is going to come in his Father's glory with his angels, and then he will reward each person according to what he has done.	
273 Deuteronomy 4.23: Be careful not to forget the covenant of the LORD your God that he made with you; do not make for yourselves an idol in the form of anything the LORD your God has forbidden.	
274 Luke 6.38: . . . For with the measure you use, it will be measured to you.	
275 2 Corinthians 5.9: So we make it our goal to please him, whether we are at home in the body or away from it.	
276 Romans 9.21: Does not the potter have the right to make out of the same lump of clay some pottery for noble purposes and some for common use?	
Week 37 and 50	**Memorise?**
277 Romans 10.11 As the Scripture says, "Anyone who trust in him will never be put to shame."	
278 Lamentations 3.40: Let us examine our ways and test them, and let us return to the LORD.	
279 Philippians 2.12-13: . . . continue to work out your salvation with fear and trembling, for it is God who works in you to will and to act according to his good purpose.	
280 1 Timothy 5.1-2: Do not rebuke an older man harshly, but exhort him as if he were your father. Treat younger men as brothers, older women as mothers, and younger women as sisters, with absolute purity.	
281 2 Thessalonians 3.16: Now may the Lord of peace himself give you peace at all times and in every way	
282 Proverbs 20.5: The purposes of a man's heart are deep waters, but a man of understanding draws them out.	
283 Galatians 5.22: But the fruit of the Spirit is love, joy, peace, patience, kindness, goodness, faithfulness, gentleness and self-control.	
284 Isaiah 55.7: Let the wicked forsake his way and the evil man his thoughts. Let him turn to the LORD and he will have mercy on him, and to our God, for he will freely pardon.	

285 Psalm 101.2: I will be careful to lead a blameless life—when will you come to me? I will walk in my house with blameless heart.	
286 Proverbs 24.17: Do not gloat when your enemy falls when he stumbles do not let your heart rejoice . . .	
287 Matthew 9.13: But go and learn what this means: 'I desire mercy, not sacrifice'.	
288 Micah 6.8: He has showed you, O man, what is good. And what does the LORD require of you? To act justly and to love mercy and to walk humbly with your God.	
Week 38 and 51	**Memorise?**
289 Titus 2.11-13: For the grace of God that brings salvation has appeared to all men. It teaches us to say "No" to ungodliness and worldly passions, and to live self-controlled, upright and godly lives in the present age, while we wait for the blessed hope—the glorious appearing of our great God and Savior, Jesus Christ . . .	
290 Matthew 5.36: And do not swear by your head, for you cannot make even one hair white or black. Simply let your 'Yes' be 'Yes,' and your 'No,' 'No'; anything beyond this comes from the evil one.	
291 Luke 22.19: And he took bread, gave thanks, and broke it, and gave it to them . . .	
292 1 Peter 4.10-12: Each one should use whatever gift he has received to serve others, faithfully administering God's grace in its various forms. If anyone speaks, he should do it as one speaking the very words of God. If anyone serves, he should do it with the strength God provides, so that in all things God may be praised through Jesus Christ	
293 Romans 14.17-18: For the kingdom of God is not a matter of eating and drinking, but of righteousness, peace and joy in the Holy Spirit, because anyone who serves Christ in this way is pleasing to God and approved by men.	
294 Romans 12.14-16: Bless those who persecute you; bless and do not curse. Rejoice with those who rejoice; mourn with those who mourn. Live in harmony with one another. Do not be proud, but be willing to associate with people of low position. Do not be conceited.	
295 Proverbs 4.5: Get wisdom, get understanding; do not forget my words or swerve from them.	
296 Ephesians 4.28: He who has been stealing must steal no longer, but must work, doing something useful with his own hands, that he may have something to share with those in need.	
297 Isaiah 58.9-10: . . . If you do away with the yoke of oppression, with the pointing finger and malicious talk, and if you spend yourselves in behalf of the hungry and satisfy the needs of the oppressed, then your light will rise in the darkness, and your night will become like the noonday.	
298 Philippians 4.7: And the peace of God, which transcends all understanding, will guard your hearts and your minds in Christ Jesus.	

	Memorise?
299 Mark 4.40: He said to his disciples, "Why are you so afraid? Do you still have no faith?"	
300 1 Corinthians 16.13: Be on your guard; stand firm in the faith; be men of courage; be strong. Do everything in love.	
Week 39 and 52	**Memorise?**
301 Romans 12.2: Do not conform any longer to the pattern of this world, but be transformed by the renewing of your mind. Then you will be able to test and approve what God's will is—his good, pleasing and perfect will.	
302 Colossians 3.5: Put to death, therefore, whatever belongs to your earthly nature; sexual immorality, impurity, lust, evil desires and greed, which is idolatry.	
303 1 Corinthians 10.13: . . . And God is faithful; he will not let you be tempted beyond what you can bear. But when you are tempted, he will also provide a way out so that you can stand up under it.	
304 Matthew 5.7: Blessed are the merciful, for they will be shown mercy.	
305 Acts 8.30-31: . . . "Do you understand what you are reading?" Phillip asked. "How can I," he said, "unless someone explains it to me?"	
306 Job 15.2-4: Would a wise man answer with empty notions or fill his belly with the hot east wind? Would he argue with useless words, with speeches that have no value? But you even undermine piety and hinder devotion to God.	
307 1 Peter 2.4-5: As you come to him, the living Stone—rejected by men but chosen by God and precious to him—you also, like living stones, are being built into a spiritual house to be a holy priesthood, offering spiritual sacrifices acceptable to God through Jesus Christ.	
308 Ephesians 6.18: And pray in the Spirit on all occasions with all kinds of prayers and requests. With this in mind, be alert and always keep on praying for all the saints.	
309 Deuteronomy 8.3: He humbled you, causing you to hunger and then feeding you with manna, which neither you nor your fathers had known, to teach you that man does not live on bread alone but on every word that comes from the mouth of the LORD.	
310 Proverbs 21.13: If a man shuts his ears to the cry of the poor, he too will cry out and not be answered.	
311 Hebrews 3.14: We have come to share in Christ if we hold firmly till the end the confidence we had at first.	
312 Ephesians 5.1-2: Be imitators of God, therefore, as dearly loved children and live a life of love, just as Christ loved us and gave himself up for us as a fragrant offering and sacrifice to God.	

PRAY FOR . . .
People you know and come into contact with, as well as . . .

A Ambulance workers Those in authority	The aged Absent friends	Alcoholics The angry	Animal workers Those who face adversity	Addicts Victims of accidents
B Business leaders Broken families	The Blind	Battered women	The broken-hearted	Bible colleges
C Couples facing marital difficulties	Children The Christian community	Clergy The childless	Child workers	Charity workers
D Divorcees The deformed Those in disgrace The destitute	Domestic workers The despised Those in distress	The disabled The depressed	Doctors and nurses People dying	Deaf and dumb Those in despair
E Educationalists	Expectant mothers	Elderly people	The exploited	Enemies
F The Frightened Farmers and Farmworkers	Family Those of other faiths The fearful	Frail Fund raisers Friends	Fathers Those without faith The forgotten	Fishermen Those in financial difficulties
G The grieving	Gang leaders	Those addicted to gambling		
H HIV/Aids The hard-hearted	Hospital workers The homeless	The hungry Those who have lost hope	Those leaving home for 1st time	The heartsore and heart-broken
I Ill people	Innocent victims			
J Juvenile delinquents	Judges and magistrates			
K				
L Lonely	Leaders	Those who have lost their homes	The lukewarm	Lepers
M Missionaries and evangelists	The military Those who mourn	Mineworkers and dangerous occupations	Those maimed by war/terrorism	Those about to get married
N Neighbours	Those in need	Nursing staff		Those in nursing homes
O Our congregation	Orphans	The overworked		
P President	People writing examinations	Police	Poor Those in pain	The persecuted
The perplexed	Politicians	Prisoners	Prayer groups	Peacemakers
Q				
R Relatives Rotary, etc	Retrenched	The rejected	Racial harmony	Refugees
S Sunday school children The saints	Sea rescue Street children	Those about to have surgery	Sexually abused Those under stress	Students The sorrowful

T Those in trouble or need Those who believe themselves failures	Those who anger us Those in mental hospitals	Those with a debilitating disease Alzheimer	People traveling Those training to be priests	Those facing temptation Those contemplating suicide
U Unemployed	Underprivileged	Unmarried mothers	The lonely and unloved	Those unhappy with their work
V People in violent relationships	Volunteer workers	Victims of violence		
W Widows	Work colleagues	Welfare organizations	Those in war zones	The wayward and wandering
X				
Y Young marrieds	Youth			
Z	Zenophobia victims			

THANKS FOR EVERYDAY THINGS

01 A friendly word	21 Church	41 Helping me to care	61 Opening my eyes	81 Shelter
02 A good laugh	22 Communications received	42 Health	62 Outings	82 Sins forgiven
03 A hot shower on a cold morning	23 Calm and stability	43 Helping me to reach out	63 Overcoming difficulties	83 Sleep
04 A job	24 Controlling my thoughts	44 Holidays	64 Peace	84 Small mercies
05 A regular income	25 Courage in times of difficulty	45 Hospitality shown to me	65 People who accept me as I am	85 Starlight
06 A roof over my head	26 Delicious smells	46 Inner conviction	66 People who make a difference	86 Strength of mind and body
07 A sense of Your presence	27 Education	47 Insights	67 Pets	87 Sunrises and sunsets
08 A serene mind	28 Enjoyable company	48 Keepng me alive	68 Physical activity	88 The ability to be fascinated
09 A wise person's counsel	29 Entertainment	49 Kindnesses received	69 Prayer	89 A loving touch
10 A word of comfort	30 Eyesight	50 Bird song	70 Recognition	90 The ability to dream
11 Absence of pain	31 Family	51 Labour saving devices	71 Relatives	91 The joy of worship
12 Achievements	32 Food	52 Love	72 Relaxation	92 The solitude of mountains
13 An interest in life	33 Forgiveness	53 Material possessions	73 Relief from anxiety	93 The changing seasons
14 An unexpected smile	34 Freedom from pain	54 Medicine	74 Resisting temptation	94 Those who cheered me up
15 Another's courage and guts	35 Freedom from fear	55 Modern technology	75 Role models	95 Times of celebration
16 Beauty	36 Friendship	56 Music	76 Safety	96 Touch, smell sound, sight, hearing
17 Bird song	37 Good government	57 My growth	77 Scenery	97 Unexpected joys
18 Birds and butterflies	38 God's supreme kindness and love	58 My talents	78 Sensible advice	98 Variety
19 Books	39 Happy things	59 Nature	79 Sensitivity	99 Warmth and shelter
20 Children	40 Health	60 New discoveries	80 Sex	100 Wonders of the universe

52 ATTRIBUTES TO CULTIVATE

As you meditate each week on one of the following, ask yourself "What can I do to be more Christ-like in thought word and deed?"

1. Honesty and humility	2. Love of neighbour	3. Detachment from worldly things	5. The gift of prayer	6. Control over my body
7. Right use of my mind	8. Peace and serenity	9. Patience under trials	10. Love of God and longing to serve Him	11. Paying attention to important details
12. Right use of gifts and talents	13. Perseverance in the faith	14. Strength to eradicate pernicious faults	15. Willingness to take up the Cross	15. A desire to help others
16. Tenderness and gentleness	17. Mastery of self	18. Diligence	19. The ability to cheer and comfort others	20. A love of Bible study
21. A passion for listening	22. Perseverance in being a good steward	23. A resolute nature	24. Avoidance of anxiety	25. An intimate loving relationship with Jesus
26. A heart that worships and praises	27. Being an example to others	28. Celebrating life's beautiful moments	29. Sacrificing my desires for a greater good	30. Being a centre of calm and stability
31. Being temperate and moderate	32. Showing appreciation for all things	33. Having the courage of my convictions	34. Rejecting hypocrisy in myself and others	35. Avoiding slackness when doing my duty
36. Giving without patronage	37. Remaining sensitive to others	38. Making the most use of my time	39. Strengthening my belief through faith and knowledge	40. Being committed to causes I believe in
41. Learning the lesson that disappointment brings	42. Discovering the values I hold most dear	43. Forgiving others, forgiving myself	44. Upholding integrity in all my dealings	45. Fighting against injustice
46. Nurturing the good within me	47. The practice of hospitality	48. Avoiding self-righteousness	49. Treasuring the sacred in everyday life	50. Acquiring wisdom
51. The imperative of love	52. Balance and mindfulness			

52 SINS TO AVOID

As you meditate each week on one of the following, pray for God's grace to show you what is the one thing you must do to grow in Christian perfection.

1. Greed	2. Envy	3. Vanity	4. Resentment	5. Anger
6. Pride	7. Faithlessness	8. Excess	9. Untruthfulness	10. Ingratitude
11. Self-righteousness	12. Disparagement	13. Negligence	14. Idolatry	15. Prodigality
16. Lukewarmness	17. Uncharitableness	18. Jealousy	19. Meanness	20. Wastefulness
21. Hypocrisy	22. Wantonness	23. Impiety	24. Dissipation	25. Covetousness
26. Blasphemy	27. Inconsideration	28. Cowardice	29. Thoughtlessness	30. Disobedience
31. Self-indulgence	32. Bullying	33. Self-importance	34. Lovelessness	35. Lack of discipline
36. Malice	37. Dishonesty	38. Boasting	39. Abuse of time, self, others	40. Judging others
41. Jealousy	42. Acrimony	43. Unkindness	44. Hard-heartedness	45. Distrust of God's word
46. Impatience	47. Causing pain	48. Complacency	49. Negligence	50. Swearing
51. Lust	52. Deceit			

The Principles of the Third Order of the Society of St Francis

Day 1—The Object

JESUS said "Very truly I tell you, unless a grain of wheat falls into the earth and dies, it remains but a single grain, but if it dies, it bears much fruit. Those who love their life lose it, and those who hate their life in this world will keep it for eternal life. *Whoever serves me must follow me, and where I am there will my servant be also.* Whoever serves me the Father will honour. John 12.24-26

Day 2—The Object cont'd

By the **example** of his own **sacrifice, JESUS** reveals *the secret of bearing fruit.* In surrendering himself to death, he becomes the source of new life. Lifted from the earth on the cross, he draws all people to himself. *Clinging to life causes life to decay,* the life that is freely given is eternal.

Day Three—The Object cont'd

JESUS calls those who would *serve him* to *follow his example* and *choose* for themselves the same path of *renunciation and sacrifice.* To those who *hear* and *obey* he promises union with God.

The object of the Society of Saint Francis is to build a community of those who accept Christ as their Lord and Master and are dedicated to him in body and spirit. They **surrender their lives to him** and to the service of his people. The Third Order of the Society consists of those who, while following the ordinary professions of life, feel called to dedicate their lives under a definite discipline and vows. They may be female or male, married or single, ordained or lay.

Day Four—The Object cont'd

When St Francis encouraged the formation of the Third Order he recognized that many are called to serve God in the spirit of **Poverty, Chastity and Obedience** in everyday life (rather than in a literal acceptance of these principles as in the vows of the Brothers and Sisters of the First and Second Orders.) The Rule of the Third Order is intended to enable the duties and conditions of daily living to be carried out in this spirit.

Day Five—The First Aim of the Order

To make our Lord known and loved everywhere.

The Order is founded on the conviction that **JESUS CHRIST** is the perfect revelation of God, that true life has been made available to us through his Incarnation and Ministry, by his Cross and Resurrection, and by the sending of the Holy Spirit. The Order believes that it is the commission of the church to make the gospel known to all and therefore **accept the duty of bringing others to know CHRIST, and of praying and working for the coming of the Kingdom of God.**

Day Six—The First Aim, cont'd

The primary aim of the tertiaries is therefore to make CHRIST known. This shapes their lives and attitudes to reflect the obedience of those whom our Lord chose to be with him and sent out as witnesses. Like them, tertiaries, by word and example bear witness to CHRIST in their own immediate environment and pray and work for the fulfillment of his commandment to make disciples of all nations.

Day Seven—The Second Aim

To spread the spirit of love and harmony

The Order sets out, in the name of **CHRIST**, to break down barriers between people and to seek equality for all.

Tertiaries accept as their second aim the spreading of a spirit of love and harmony among all people. **They are pledged to fight against the ignorance, pride and prejudice that breeds injustice or partiality because of distinctions of race, sex, colour, class, creed, status or education.**

Day Eight—The Second Aim, cont'd

Tertiaries fight against all such injustice in the name of **CHRIST** in whom there can be neither Jew nor Greek, slave nor free, male nor female, for in him all are one. Their chief object is to reflect that openness to all which was characteristic of Jesus. **This can only be achieved in a spirit of chastity which sees others as belonging to God and not as a means of self-fulfillment.**

Day Nine—The Second Aim, cont'd

Tertiaries are prepared not only to speak out for social justice and international peace, but in their own lives, cheerfully facing any scorn or persecution to which this may lead.

Day Ten—The Third Aim

To live simply

The first Christians surrendered completely to our Lord and recklessly gave all that they had, offering the world a new vision of a society in which a fresh attitude was taken towards material possessions. This vision was renewed by St Francis when he chose Lady Poverty as his bride, desiring that all barriers set up by privilege based on wealth should be overcome by love. This is the inspiration for the aim of the Society, to live simply.

Day Eleven—The Third Aim, cont'd

Tertiaries, though they possess property and earn money to support themselves and their families, show themselves true followers of Christ and Saint Francis by their readiness to live simply and to share with others. They recognise that some of their members may be called to a literal following of Saint Francis in a life of extreme simplicity. **All, however, accept that they avoid luxury and waste**, and regard their possessions as being in held in trust for God.

Day Twelve—The Third Aim, cont'd

Personal spending is limited to what is necessary for the health and wellbeing of themselves and their dependants. They aim to stay free from all attachment to wealth, keeping themselves constantly aware of the poverty in the world and its claim on them. Tertiaries are concerned more for the generosity that gives all, rather than the value of poverty in itself. In this way they reflect in spirit the acceptance of Jesus' challenge to sell all, give to the poor, and follow him.

Day Thirteen—The Three Ways of Service

Tertiaries desire to be conformed to the image of Jesus Christ, whom they serve in the three ways of **Prayer, Study and Work. In the life of the Order as a whole, these three ways must each find full and balanced expression,** but it is not to be expected that all members devote themselves equally to each of them. Each individual's service varies according to his/her abilities and circumstances, yet the member's personal rule of life includes each of the three ways.

Day Fourteen—The First Way of Service—Prayer

Tertiaries seek to live in an atmosphere of praise and prayer. They aim to be constantly aware of God's presence, so that they may indeed pray without ceasing. Their ever-deepening devotion to the indwelling Christ is a source of strength and joy. **It is Christ's love that inspires them to service and strengthens them for sacrifice.**

Day Fifteen—The First Way of Service, cont'd

The heart of their prayer is the Eucharist, in which they share with other Christians the renewal of their union with their Lord and Saviour in his sacrifice, remembering his death and receiving his spiritual food.

Day Sixteen—The First Way of Service, cont'd

Tertiaries recognise the power of intercessory prayer for furthering the purposes of God's kingdom, and therefore seek a deepening communion with God in personal devotion, and constantly intercede for the needs of his church and his world. Those who have much time at their disposal give prayer a large part of their daily lives. Those with less time must not fail to see the importance of prayer and to guard the time they have allotted to it from interruption. Lastly, tertiaries are encouraged to avail themselves of the sacrament of Reconciliation, through which the burden of past sin and failure is lifted and peace and hope restored.

Day Seventeen—The Second Way of Service—Study.

"And this is eternal life: that they may know you the only true God, and Jesus Christ whom you have sent." John 17.3

True knowledge is knowledge of God. **Tertiaries therefore give priority to devotional study of scripture** as one of the chief means of attaining the knowledge of God which leads to eternal life.

Day Eighteen—The Second Way of Service, cont'd.

As well as the devotional study of Scripture, all recognise **their Christian responsibility to pursue other branches of study, both sacred and secular.** In particular there are membersof the Third Order who accept the duty of contributing, through their research and writing, to a better understanding of the church's mission in the world: the application of Christian principles to the use and distribution of wealth; questions concerning justice and peace; and all other questions concerning the life of faith.

Day Nineteen—The Third Way of Service—Work

Jesus took on himself the form of a servant. **He came not to be served but to serve.** He went about doing good: healing the sick, preaching good news to the poor, and binding up the broken-hearted.

Day Twenty—The Third Way of Service, cont'd

Tertiaries endeavour to serve others in active work. **They try to find expression for each of the three aims of the Order in their lives,** and whenever possible actively help others who are engaged in similar work. The chief form of service which Tertiaries have to offer is to reflect the love of Christ, who in his beauty and power, is the inspiration and joy of their lives.

Day Twenty One—The Three Notes of the Order

Humility, love and joy are the three notes which mark the lives of Tertiaries. When these characteristics are evident throughout the Order, its work will be fruitful. **Without them, all of them, all that it attempts will be in vain.**

Day Twenty Two—The First Note—Humility

Tertiaries always keep before them the example of Christ, who emptied himself, taking the form of a servant, and who, on the last day of his life, humbly washed his disciples' feet. They likewise seek to serve one another with humility.

Day Twenty Three—The First Note, cont'd

Humility confesses that we have nothing that we have not received and admits the fact of our insufficiency and our dependence upon God. It is the basis of Christian virtues. Saint Bernard of Clairvaux said, "No spiritual house can stand for a moment except on the foundation of humility." It is the first condition of a joyful life within any community.

Day Twenty Four—The First Note, cont'd

The faults tertiaries see in others are the subject of prayer rather than criticism. They take care to cast out the beam from their own eye before offering to remove the speck from another's They are ready to accept the lowest place when asked and to volunteer to take it. Nevertheless, when asked to undertake work of which they feel unworthy or incapable they do not shrink from it on the grounds of humility, but confidently attempt it through the power that is made perfect in weakness.

Day Twenty Five—The Second Note—Love

JESUS said, "I give you a new commandment: love one another. Just as I have loved you, you also should love one another. By this everyone will know that you are my disciples, if you have love for one another." John 13. 34-35

Love is the distinguishing feature of all true disciples of Christ who wish to dedicate themselves to him as his servants.

Day Twenty Six—The Second Note, cont'd

Therefore, tertiaries seek to love all those to whom they are bound by ties of family or friendship. Their love for them increases as their love for Christ grows deeper.

They have a special love and affection for members of the Third Order, praying for each other individually and seeking to grow in that love. They are on their guard against anything which might injure this love, and they seek reconciliation with those from whom they are estranged. They seek the same love for those with whom they have little natural affinity, for this kind of love is not a welling up of emotion, but is a bond founded in their common union with Christ.

Day Twenty Seven—The Second Note, cont'd

The Third Order is Christian community whose members, although varied in race, education and character, are bound into a living whole through the love they share in Christ. This unity of all who believe in him will become, as our Lord intended, a witness to the world of his divine mission.

In their relationship with those outside the Order, tertiaries show the same Christ-like love, and gladly give of themselves, remembering that love is measured by sacrifice.

Day Twenty Eight—The Third Note—Joy

Tertiaries, rejoicing in the Lord always, show in their lives the grace and beauty of divine joy. They remember that they follow the Son of Man, who came eating and drinking, who loved the birds and the flowers, who blessed little children, who was a friend of tax collectors and sinners, who sat at the tables of both the rich and the poor. Tertiaries delight in fun and laughter, rejoicing in God's world, its beauty and its living creatures, calling nothing common or unclean. They mix freely with all people, ready to bind up the broken-hearted, and to bring joy into the lives of others. They carry within them an inner peace and happiness which others may perceive, even if they do not know its source.

Day Twenty Nine, cont'd

This joy is a divine gift, coming from union with God in Christ. It is still there even in times of darkness and difficulty, giving cheerful courage in the face of disappointment, and an inward serenity and confidence through sickness and suffering. Those who possess it can rejoice in weakness, insults, hardship, and persecutions for Christ's sake, for when they are weak, then they are strong.

Day Thirty—The Three Notes

The humility, love and joy which mark the lives of tertiaries are all God given graces. They can never be obtained by human effort. They are gifts of the Holy Spirit. The purpose of Christ is to work miracles through people who are willing to be emptied of self and to surrender to him. They then become channels of grace through whom his mighty work is done.

Index of biblical quotations

Quoted sources	Where found Biblical helps	Type
EXODUS **4:12** **34:6-7**	 Week 47 Week 3	 *WORDS OF ENCOURAGEMENT* *WORDS OF ENCOURAGEMENT*
LEVITICUS 25:43	 008	 RIGHT ACTION
NUMBERS 6:24-26 12:6	 010 229	 RIGHT ATTITUDE LEARNING/LISTENING
DEUTERONOMY 4:23 6:5 6:6 8:3 **20.4** **28:2** 30:19	 273 095 003 309 Week 23 Week 28 250	 REPENTANCE/RENEWAL LEARNING/LISTENING FAITH AND FRIENDSHIP PRAISE AND PRAYER *WORDS OF ENCOURAGEMENT* *WORDS OF ENCOURAGEMENT* RIGHT AVOIDANCE
JOSHUA **1.9** 24:14	 Week 29 231	 *WORDS OF ENCOURAGEMENT* PRAISE AND PRAYER
1 SAMUEL 2:3 **12:24**	 198 Week 49	 RIGHT AVOIDANCE *WORDS OF ENCOURAGEMENT*
2 KINGS 20:5	 069	 REPENTANCE/RENEWAL
NEHEMIAH 9:17	 034	 RIGHT ATTITUDE

JOB		
4:6	142	Right Avoidance
5:8	180	Right Avoidance
5:17	220	Right Avoidance
6:14	098	Right Action
15:2-4	306	Right Avoidance
33:4	Week 43	*WORDS OF ENCOURAGEMENT*
34:4	218	Right Avoidance
PSALMS		
1: 1-2	169	Learning/Listening
9:1-2	027	Prayer and praise
12:2	062	Right Avoidance
16:11	Week 50	*WORDS OF ENCOURAGEMENT*
18:30	129	thanks and trust
19:1	121	Learning/Listening
19:8	149	Learning/Listening
23:1-3	211	Faith and Friendship
23:6	Week 38	*WORDS OF ENCOURAGEMENT*
27:4	265	Praise and prayer
27:14	Week 26	*WORDS OF ENCOURAGEMENT*
32:5	147	Repentance/renewal
32:8	111	thanks and trust
35:18	079	thanks and trust
36: 9	Week 39	*WORDS OF ENCOURAGEMENT*
37:4	Week 25	*WORDS OF ENCOURAGEMENT*
37:7	Week 19	*WORDS OF ENCOURAGEMENT*
37:39	Week 20	*WORDS OF ENCOURAGEMENT*
37:40	085	thanks and trust
47:7	159	Praise and prayer
62:12	Week 1	*WORDS OF ENCOURAGEMENT*
63:8	227	Faith and Friendship
73:23-24	Week 33	*WORDS OF ENCOURAGEMENT*
81:10	Week 30	*WORDS OF ENCOURAGEMENT*
81:11-12	045	Learning/Listening
84:11	Week 44	*WORDS OF ENCOURAGEMENT*
86:15	Week 45	*WORDS OF ENCOURAGEMENT*
101:2	285	Discipline/ Discipleship
103:1	123	Praise and prayer
106:1-2	201	thanks and trust
106:3	054	Right Attitude
119:1	Week 36	*WORDS OF ENCOURAGEMENT*
119:2	Week 52	*WORDS OF ENCOURAGEMENT*
119:24	163	Faith and Friendship
119:132-133	Week 51	*WORDS OF ENCOURAGEMENT*

119:37	116	RIGHT AVOIDANCE
119:78	183	LEARNING/LISTENING
119:133	153	DISCIPLINE/ DISCIPLESHIP
119:165	Week 40	*WORDS OF ENCOURAGEMENT*
121.7	Week 24	*WORDS OF ENCOURAGEMENT*
127:1	157	REPENTANCE/RENEWAL
131:1-2	127	FAITH AND FRIENDSHIP
128:1-2	Week 27	*WORDS OF ENCOURAGEMENT*
130.5	Week 48	*WORDS OF ENCOURAGEMENT*
135.14	Week 32	*WORDS OF ENCOURAGEMENT*
138.3	Week 5	*WORDS OF ENCOURAGEMENT*
139:23	240	RIGHT AVOIDANCE
142.3	Week 41	*WORDS OF ENCOURAGEMENT*
145.17-18	Week 46	*WORDS OF ENCOURAGEMENT*
146:2	001	PRAISE AND PRAYER
PROVERBS		
1.33	245	LEARNING/LISTENING
3:5	235	THANKS AND TRUST
3:5	Week 4	*WORDS OF ENCOURAGEMENT*
3:27	022	RIGHT ACTION
4:1-2	049	LEARNING/LISTENING
4:4	177	DISCIPLINE/ DISCIPLESHIP
4:5	295	LEARNING/LISTENING
4:13-14	068	RIGHT ATTITUDE
6:6	214	RIGHT ACTION
6:16-19	112	RIGHT ATTITUDE
11:1	114	RIGHT AVOIDANCE
11:12	216	RIGHT AVOIDANCE
11:24	178	RIGHT ATTITUDE
12:15	225	LEARNING/LISTENING
12:18	182	RIGHT ATTITUDE
12:20	134	RIGHT ATTITUDE
12:25	082	RIGHT ATTITUDE
14:21	072	RIGHT ATTITUDE
15:28	232	RIGHT ATTITUDE
16:7-8	044	RIGHT ACTION
16:24	014	RIGHT ATTITUDE
17:22	158	RIGHT ATTITUDE
19:11	032	RIGHT AVOIDANCE
19:17	262	RIGHT ATTITUDE
19:21	243	FAITH AND FRIENDSHIP
20:3	154	RIGHT AVOIDANCE
20:5	282	RIGHT ATTITUDE
20:27	199	LEARNING/LISTENING

21:21	108	RIGHT ATTITUDE
21:13	310	RIGHT ACTION
24:17	286	RIGHT AVOIDANCE
24:29	188	RIGHT AVOIDANCE
25:6-7	170	RIGHT AVOIDANCE
25:28	196	RIGHT AVOIDANCE
28:20	193	FAITH AND FRIENDSHIP
30:5-6	077	LEARNING/LISTENING
30:32	038	RIGHT ATTITUDE
31:8	106	RIGHT ACTION
ECCLESIASTES		
5:1-2	119	PRAISE AND PRAYER
8.5	Week 7	*WORDS OF ENCOURAGEMENT*
9.7	Week 11	*WORDS OF ENCOURAGEMENT*
11.1	Week 8	*WORDS OF ENCOURAGEMENT*
12:14	140	RIGHT ATTITUDE
ISAIAH		
1:18	035	FAITH AND FRIENDSHIP
26:4	061	THANKS AND TRUST
30:21	209	PRAISE AND PRAYER
40.29	Week 16	*WORDS OF ENCOURAGEMENT*
41:10	173	FAITH AND FRIENDSHIP
41:28	254	RIGHT ACTION
42.16	Week 22	*WORDS OF ENCOURAGEMENT*
42:20	026	RIGHT ACTION
44.22	Week 12	*WORDS OF ENCOURAGEMENT*
44.28	Week 21	*WORDS OF ENCOURAGEMENT*
55:7	284	RIGHT AVOIDANCE
58:9-10	297	REPENTANCE/RENEWAL
JEREMIAH		
7:23	206	RIGHT ACTION
17:7-8	021	THANKS AND TRUST
17:9	252	RIGHT ATTITUDE
22:3	260	RIGHT AVOIDANCE
29:11	247	THANKS AND TRUST
39:12	148	RIGHT AVOIDANCE
LAMENTATIONS		
3:40	278	RIGHT ATTITUDE
4:4	258	RIGHT ACTION
3:25-26	103	REPENTANCE/RENEWAL
DANIEL		
4:27	120	RIGHT ATTITUDE
6:10	179	THANKS AND TRUST

HOSEA		
10:12	090	RIGHT ATTITUDE
12:6	126	RIGHT ATTITUDE
JOEL		
2:13	087	REPENTANCE/RENEWAL
AMOS		
5:4	Week 14	*WORDS OF ENCOURAGEMENT*
MICAH		
6:8	288	RIGHT ACTION
NAHUM		
ZEPHANIAH		
3.17	Week 18	*WORDS OF ENCOURAGEMENT*
MATTHEW		
5:5	256	RIGHT ATTITUDE
5:7	304	RIGHT ATTITUDE
5:8	171	REPENTANCE/RENEWAL
5.14	092	RIGHT ACTION
5.16	036	RIGHT ACTION
5:22	080	RIGHT AVOIDANCE
5:36	290	RIGHT ATTITUDE
5:41	076	RIGHT ACTION
5:42	084	RIGHT ACTION
5:44-45	071	PRAISE AND PRAYER
5:48	213	REPENTANCE/RENEWAL
6:1	203	DISCIPLINE/ DISCIPLESHIP
6:3-4	186	RIGHT ACTION
6:7-8	099	PRAISE AND PRAYER
6:14-15	194	RIGHT ATTITUDE
6:19-21	143	DISCIPLINE/ DISCIPLESHIP
6:31-33	205	THANKS AND TRUST
6:34	164	RIGHT AVOIDANCE
7:2	018	RIGHT AVOIDANCE
7:7	165	LEARNING/LISTENING
7:11	185	THANKS AND TRUST
7:12	208	RIGHT ATTITUDE
9:13	287	LEARNING/LISTENING
11:28	255	FAITH AND FRIENDSHIP
11:29	105	LEARNING/LISTENING
12:25	089	FAITH AND FRIENDSHIP
12:34-35	200	RIGHT ACTION
15:11	104	RIGHT AVOIDANCE
16:26-27	272	RIGHT ACTION

17.20	065	FAITH AND FRIENDSHIP
18:6	217	REPENTANCE/RENEWAL
19:19	040	RIGHT ATTITUDE
21:22	019	PRAISE AND PRAYER
22:21	224	RIGHT ACTION
23:12	226	RIGHT ATTITUDE
25:35	124	RIGHT ACTION
25:40	222	RIGHT ACTION
MARK		
3:35	236	RIGHT ACTION
4:40	299	FAITH AND FRIENDSHIP
7:21	052	RIGHT AVOIDANCE
10:21	237	FAITH AND FRIENDSHIP
16:15	125	DISCIPLINE/ DISCIPLESHIP
LUKE		
2:19	263	LEARNING/LISTENING
3:9	025	DISCIPLINE/ DISCIPLESHIP
6:12	073	PRAYER AND PRAISE
6.27-28	228	RIGHT ATTITUDE
6:31	078	PRAYER AND PRAISE
6:35	271	THANKS AND TRUST
6:38	274	RIGHT ACTION
6:36-38	050	RIGHT ACTION
6:41	030	PRAYER AND PRAISE
9:47-48	097	DISCIPLINE/ DISCIPLESHIP
10:35	174	PRAISE AND PRAYER
11:17	135	FAITH AND FRIENDSHIP
13:24	075	DISCIPLINE/ DISCIPLESHIP
14:27	161	DISCIPLINE/ DISCIPLESHIP
16:10	167	THANKS AND TRUST
17:10	110	RIGHT ACTION
18:1	175	PRAISE AND PRAYER
22:19	291	THANKS AND TRUST
JOHN		
6:27	195	PRAISE AND PRAYER
7:16-17	063	LEARNING/LISTENING
12.26	Week 6	*WORDS OF ENCOURAGEMENT*
13:34	146	PRAISE AND PRAYER
14:6	215	LEARNING/LISTENING
14.14	Week 10	*WORDS OF ENCOURAGEMENT*
14:27	138	RIGHT ACTION
15.5	Week 42	*WORDS OF ENCOURAGEMENT*
15:13	011	THANKS AND TRUST

ACTS		
8:30-31	305	Learning/Listening
17:28	047	Discipline/ Discipleship
20:35	066	Right Action
ROMANS		
1:16	055	Faith and Friendship
2.6	166	Right Attitude
4.3	Week 34	*WORDS OF ENCOURAGEMENT*
6:12	264	Right Avoidance
6:23	007	Repentance/renewal
7:20	266	Right Avoidance
8:1-2	269	Faith and Friendship
8:18	257	Repentance/renewal
8:26	181	Praise and prayer
8:28	191	Discipline/ Discipleship
8:35	139	thanks and trust
9:21	276	Right Avoidance
10:11	277	thanks and trust
10:17	009	Learning/Listening
12:1	233	Discipline/ Discipleship
12:2	301	Repentance/renewal
12:9-11	234	Right Attitude
12:14-16	294	Right Action
12:17-18	150	Right Action
12:21	100	Right Avoidance
14:7-8	190	Right Action
14:12	020	Right Attitude
14:13	086	Right Avoidance
14:17-18	293	Praise and prayer
14:19	058	Right Avoidance
15:1-2	048	Right Attitude
1 CORINTHANS		
4:2	067	Discipline/ Discipleship
4:12-13	253	Discipline/ Discipleship
7.20		Thought for the day
10:24	042	Right Action
10:13	303	thanks and trust
10:31	041	thanks and trust
13.4-7	244	Right Action
13:11	162	Right Avoidance
14:12	017	Discipline/ Discipleship
14:15	043	Praise and prayer
16:13	300	Right Avoidance

2 CORINTHIANS		
4:2	096	RIGHT AVOIDANCE
4:8-10	219	THANKS AND TRUST
5:9	275	DISCIPLINE/ DISCIPLESHIP
6: 4 . . . 7	210	RIGHT AVOIDANCE
9:6-7	248	RIGHT ATTITUDE
9.8	Week 37	*WORDS OF ENCOURAGEMENT*
9:10-11	204	RIGHT ACTION
GALATIANS		
4:6	151	FAITH AND FRIENDSHIP
5:22	283	PRAISE AND PRAYER
6.9	Week 13	*WORDS OF ENCOURAGEMENT*
EPHESIANS		
3:20-21	057	DISCIPLINE/ DISCIPLESHIP
4:22-24	184	RIGHT AVOIDANCE
4:25-27	202	RIGHT ATTITUDE
4:28	296	RIGHT ACTION
4:29	024	RIGHT AVOIDANCE
4:31-32	130	RIGHT AVOIDANCE
5:1-2	312	RIGHT ATTITUDE
5:15-17	132	RIGHT AVOIDANCE
5:19-20	113	FAITH AND FRIENDSHIP
6.18	308	RIGHT ACTION
PHILLIPPIANS		
1:27	083	FAITH AND FRIENDSHIP
2:10-11	221	PRAISE AND PRAYER
2:12-13	279	REPENTANCE/RENEWAL
2:14-15	005	DISCIPLINE/ DISCIPLESHIP
4.5	Week 31	*WORDS OF ENCOURAGEMENT*
4.6	Week 9	*WORDS OF ENCOURAGEMENT*
4:7	298	RIGHT AVOIDANCE
4:8	109	REPENTANCE/RENEWAL
4:13	241	REPENTANCE/RENEWAL
COLOSSIANS		
1:9	141	PRAYER AND PRAISE
3:5	302	RIGHT AVOIDANCE
3:8	242	RIGHT AVOIDANCE
3:12-14	004	RIGHT ATTITUDE
3:15	031	THANKS AND TRUST
3:23	122	RIGHT ATTITUDE
4:2	261	PRAISE AND PRAYER
4:5-6	094	RIGHT ATTITUDE

1 THESSALONIANS		
4:1	267	LEARNING/LISTENING
4.3	Week 2	*WORDS OF ENCOURAGEMENT*
4:7-8	238	RIGHT AVOIDANCE
5:14-15	246	RIGHT ACTION
5:16-18	155	THANKS AND TRUST
2 THESSALONIANS		
2.16-17	Week 15	*WORDS OF ENCOURAGEMENT*
3:16	281	FAITH AND FRIENDSHIP
1 TIMOTHY		
5:1-2	280	RIGHT ACTION
5:8	128	RIGHT ACTION
6:6-7	051	THANKS AND TRUST
6:10	160	RIGHT ACTION
6.12	Week 17	*WORDS OF ENCOURAGEMENT*
2 TIMOTHY		
1:7	223	DISCIPLINE/ DISCIPLESHIP
2:15-16	192	RIGHT ATTITUDE
2:24	156	RIGHT ACTION
3:2-5	033	REPENTANCE/RENEWAL
3:16-17	023	LEARNING/LISTENING
4:3-4	133	LEARNING/LISTENING
TITUS		
1:7-8	176	RIGHT ACTION
2:11-13	289	DISCIPLINE/ DISCIPLESHIP
3:1-2	102	RIGHT ATTITUDE
HEBREWS		
2:1	115	LEARNING/LISTENING
3:12	107	FAITH AND FRIENDSHIP
3:14	311	FAITH AND FRIENDSHIP
4:16	259	THANKS AND TRUST
10:24	002	RIGHT ACTION
11:6	013	FAITH AND FRIENDSHIP
12:14	118	RIGHT ACTION
13:1-2	212	RIGHT ATTITUDE
13:4	230	RIGHT ACTION
13:5	197	REPENTANCE/RENEWAL
13:15	145	PRAISE AND PRAYER
13:16	144	RIGHT ACTION
13:17	046	RIGHT AVOIDANCE

JAMES		
1:2-4	039	FAITH AND FRIENDSHIP
1:6-7	187	REPENTANCE/RENEWAL
1:13-14	059	REPENTANCE/RENEWAL
1:17-18	172	RIGHT ACTION
1:19	029	LEARNING/LISTENING
1:26-27	152	RIGHT ATTITUDE
2:15-16	270	RIGHT ATTITUDE
2:23	189	FAITH AND FRIENDSHIP
3:16-17	239	REPENTANCE/RENEWAL
3:18	028	RIGHT AVOIDANCE
4:2-3	093	PRAISE AND PRAYER
4:7	131	REPENTANCE/RENEWAL
4:8	074	RIGHT AVOIDANCE
4:11-12	006	RIGHT AVOIDANCE
4:17	037	REPENTANCE/RENEWAL
5:9	136	RIGHT AVOIDANCE
5:16	053	PRAISE AND PRAYER
1 PETER		
1.13	Week 35	*WORDS OF ENCOURAGEMENT*
1:14-16	091	DISCIPLINE/ DISCIPLESHIP
1:22	056	RIGHT ATTITUDE
2:1	064	RIGHT AVOIDANCE
2:4-5	307	DISCIPLINE/ DISCIPLESHIP
2:12	168	RIGHT ACTION
3:9	012	RIGHT AVOIDANCE
3:17	117	DISCIPLINE/ DISCIPLESHIP
4:10-12	292	RIGHT ATTITUDE
5:7	249	DISCIPLINE/ DISCIPLESHIP
2 PETER		
1:5-7	268	RIGHT ATTITUDE
3:14	137	REPENTANCE/RENEWAL
1 JOHN		
1:6-7	015	REPENTANCE/RENEWAL
1:9-10	081	REPENTANCE/RENEWAL
2:3-4	207	DISCIPLINE/ DISCIPLESHIP
3:17	060	RIGHT ACTION
3:18	088	RIGHT ACTION
4:7-8	070	RIGHT ACTION
4.11	016	RIGHT ACTION
5:14-15	251	PRAISE AND PRAYER
REVELATION		
7:11-12	101	THANKS AND TRUST

SPIRITUAL FITNESS SCORECARD
Table 1
WEEK'S TOTAL SCORE

Add together each week's totals under **God** and **Neighbour.** Note your weekly score with a dot and join with a line. Try to do better each quarter.

% FIRST AND SECOND QUARTER

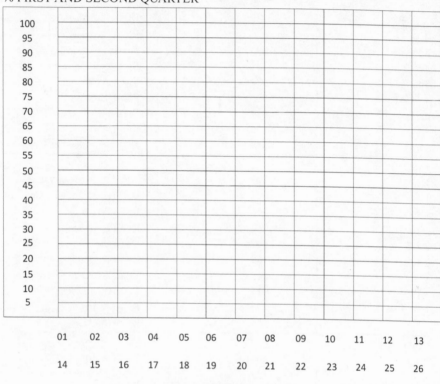

WEEKS

% THIRD AND FOURTH QUARTER

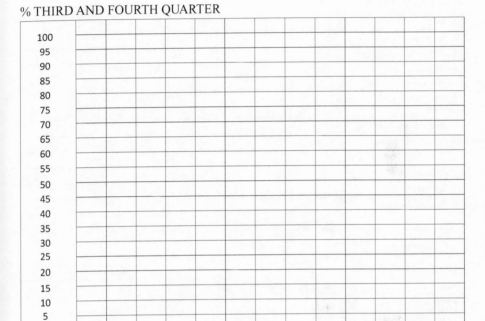

WEEKS

Table 2
LOVING GOD AND NEIGHBOUR: COMPARATIVE SCORES

In both sections below—Ψ Relationship with God; and ☺ Relationship with your neighbour—you can score a maximum of 60 points each week. Examine where, with God's help, you need to improve. Circle your lowest score.

FIRST QUARTER

WEEK	1	2	3	4	5	6	7	8	9	10	11	12	13
Ψ Prayer and praise													
Ψ Faith and friendship													
Ψ Discipline and discipleship													
Ψ Repentance and renewal													
Ψ Learning and listening													
Ψ Thanks and Trust													
Sub-total:													
☺ Right action													
☺ Right attitude													
☺ Right avoidance													
Sub-total:													

SECOND QUARTER

WEEK	14	15	16	17	18	19	20	21	22	23	24	25	26
Ψ Prayer and praise													
Ψ Faith and friendship													
Ψ Discipline and discipleship													
Ψ Repentance and renewal													
Ψ Learning and listening													
Ψ Thanks and Trust													
Sub-total:													
☺ Right action													
☺ Right attitude													
☺ Right avoidance													
Sub-total:													

THIRD QUARTER

WEEK	27	28	29	30	31	32	33	34	35	36	37	38	39
Ψ Prayer and praise													
Ψ Faith and friendship													
Ψ Discipline and discipleship													
Ψ Repentance and renewal													
Ψ Learning and listening													
Ψ Thanks and Trust													
Sub-total:													
☺ Right action													
☺ Right attitude													
☺ Right avoidance													
Sub-total:													

FOURTH QUARTER

WEEK	40	41	42	43	44	45	46	47	48	49	50	51	52
Ψ Prayer and praise													
Ψ Faith and friendship													
Ψ Discipline and discipleship													
Ψ Repentance and renewal													
Ψ Learning and listening													
Ψ Thanks and Trust													
Sub-total:													
☺ Right action													
☺ Right attitude													
☺ Right avoidance													
Sub-total:													

Table 3

PERSEVERANCE RATING %—AND DAILY REVIEW

Score your weekly perseverance rating. Are you enjoying the process?

% FIRST AND SECOND QUARTER

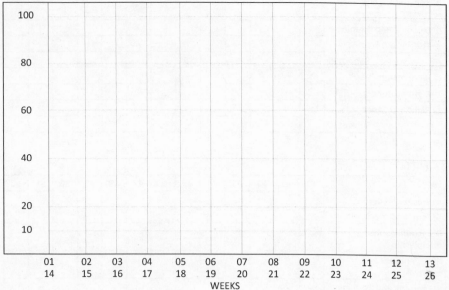

% THIRD AND FOURTH QUARTER

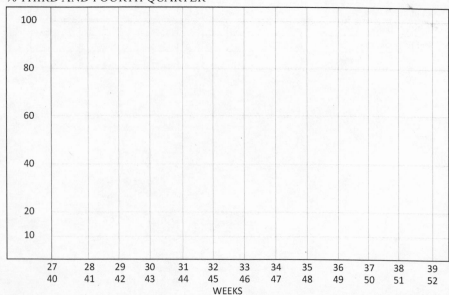